A DIETITIAN'S CANCER STORY

*Information and Inspiration for
Recovery and Healing from a
3-Time Cancer Survivor*

Fifth Edition

**By
Diana Dyer, MS, RD**

**Swan Press
PO Box 130221
Ann Arbor, MI 48113**

The information presented in this booklet describes the author's personal recovery path from her most recent cancer occurrence. It is not intended to be individualized medical or nutritional advice. Please discuss your own needs and choices for cancer treatment, recovery, and optimal wellness with your health care professionals.

ISBN 0-9667238-1-3
Library of Congress Catalog Card Number 99-90175

First printing, June 1997.
Second printing, July 1997.
Third printing, September 1997.
Fourth printing, April 1998.
Fifth printing, February 1999.

Cover design by Janus Winger, Janus Productions.
Photography by Eric Dyer
Printing by Baker Johnson, Inc, Dexter, MI

To my family
whose continuous love is the reason I did not give up
after my third cancer diagnosis

❧ TABLE OF CONTENTS ❧

❦ FOREWORD ❦

* * * * * * * * * * * * * * *

As a three-time cancer survivor as well as a health care professional, Diana Dyer offers unique perspectives on various complementary approaches to improve the quality of life in cancer patients. These approaches include lifestyle changes such as diet, exercise, meditation, as well as other techniques that should be viewed not as alternatives to conventional medicine, but rather as complementary. Furthermore, these strategies may be of value not only during the active treatment of cancer, but also during the period of recovery. By becoming active participants in these lifestyle changes, as Diana has done, cancer survivors can better regain control of their lives and improve its quality. The information in this booklet should be valuable to cancer survivors and their families.

Max Wicha, MD
Director, The University of Michigan's Comprehensive Cancer Center
Ann Arbor, Michigan

* * * * * * * * * *

COMMENTS

A sampling of comments I have received from individuals after attending my public speaking presentations, watching my MSNBC TV appearance, or reading my booklet.

****

"Because of my family history of breast cancer, I don't know what the future will bring, and frankly, I am sometimes frightened. But what has amazed me is the large number of women I have met who have experienced this illness and how they are LIVING! I really appreciated the opportunity to hear you speak. Thank you for sharing your journey."

"Our group has never given anyone else a standing ovation!"

"I was very touched and motivated by your story."

"One can't help being impressed with your interesting and informative booklet which catches the poignancy of your cancer experiences and life changes."

"Your life story is an inspiration to us all. You truly spoke to my heart."

"Your talk was one of the very best programs we have ever had presented."

"Saw you on TV (MSNBC). You were wonderful and inspiring. Thank you!"

"Thank you for your valuable information. I truly believe you are right."

"Thank you for the efforts you are making to help us. Keep up the good work."

"You are giving cancer survivors real hope. Thank you for reaching out."

"I would just like to say how interesting I found your television appearance today. It was refreshing to watch someone so down to earth and pleasant, rather than a "know-it-all" or "super-person" like so many. No doubt, your practicality has helped you to get through your ordeals."

****

❦ PREFACE FOR THE 5th EDITION ❦

My vision for the distribution of *A Dietitian's Cancer Story* has been to have it available in cancer centers across the country to be *given* to cancer patients. I wrote this book to be just what I wish my own cancer center would have given me when I started asking the question, "What else can I be doing to help with my recovery?" It is a concise guide to strategies that may help enhance the benefit of conventional cancer therapies. It also helps a newly diagnosed patient learn various techniques for becoming an equal partner in his or her cancer care and an informed consumer of complementary medicine.

Bulk pricing is available for quantity orders of my book. One cancer center has already bought enough for their patients to have an individual copy. Memorial gift funds were used to purchase these books, which was very meaningful to me.

A significant percentage of the proceeds from the sale of my books to cancer centers will be given to non-profit organizations. I will focus on organizations with a commitment to funding projects that increase our understanding of the nutrition and cancer relationship or preserve habitats on our fragile, precious planet containing plants that may hold the key to curing cancer.

After reading this book, if you believe you would have benefited by receiving it as educational material from your own cancer center, please tell someone there. The Registered Dietitian, the Clinical Nurse Specialist, the Education Coordinator, your physician, and the Cancer Center Administrator would all be appropriate health care professionals with whom to share your request.

In this edition, I have done some updates, added an extensive chapter containing tips for eating away from home, and made the book and print size larger, thus easier to read. I hope you find both information and inspiration in my book so that your cancer recovery journey is easier than mine was.

With best wishes,

Diana Dyer
February 9, 1999

❖ PREFACE TO THE 4TH EDITION ❖

So much has happened in my life during the past year since *The Detroit Free Press* published an article about my cancer recovery. I was invited to be on national TV, interviewed by many newspapers, was the invited keynote speaker for a "Race for the Cure", invited to speak to numerous cancer survivor groups, professional conferences for various health care professionals, and Medical Grand Rounds at major medical centers, along with being honored by my state professional organization (Michigan Dietetic Association) with its Individual Public Relations Award. In addition, I've had the opportunity to meet Jane Brody, author and health writer for The New York Times, and, I have received a hand-written note from Dr. Bernie Siegel, author of *Love, Medicine, and Miracles.* Amazement is an understatement!

However, writing and revising this booklet, along with mailing it out to each of you who have ordered it, have given me the greatest sense of both pleasure and contentment. I thank all of my readers, whom I think of as new friends, for the constant support and encouragement that so many of you have sent to me via telephone calls, letters, E-mail, and prayers. I also admire all of you and encourage you to start writing and speaking of your own inspirational stories that you have so openly told me.

I would like to share the quote that I usually use to end my speaking presentations. It so clearly expresses my sense of amazement and wonder at what has happened to me after my latest cancer diagnosis:

"Every journey has a secret destination of which the traveler is unaware".

• Martin Buber

My hope for you is that your own cancer journey will also lead you to unexpected, but surprisingly wonderful, people, places, and opportunities.

With warmest regards,

Diana Dyer
April 28, 1998

The idea for this book was born after one of those "defining moments" in my life. On April 8, 1997, *The Detroit Free Press* published an article entitled "Nutrition vs. Cancer" in which my recovery from a childhood cancer, neuroblastoma, and two separate breast cancers, at ages 34 and 45, was highlighted. In addition to providing an overview of current knowledge, guidelines, and research evaluating the nutrition and cancer connections, the article discussed the changes that I, as a Registered Dietitian, have made in my diet and lifestyle to minimize the risk of cancer recurrence after my second breast cancer. I did have a mastectomy and chemotherapy with each breast cancer. However, **I have chosen to recover from my second breast cancer very differently from my first one by making significant changes in both my diet and lifestyle,** many of which fall under the umbrella term of "alternative/complementary medicine".

When the *Detroit Free Press'* medical writer, Pat Anstett, suggested my telephone number be included in the article, I could not foresee why she thought that would be necessary. However, my phone began ringing before 9 AM the morning the article was published and continued almost non-stop for months following the article's distribution to newspapers throughout the country over the Knight-Ridder wire service. Additionally, the article has been clipped and sent to friends and relatives from all sections of the U.S., Canada, and at least 6 other countries that I have been told about. Although most of the articles reprinted in other newspapers did not publish my telephone number, people were creative, found my number, and called. I now truly understand the "power of the written word"! And people are still calling a full 2 years later!

The responses to this article ranged from simple "Congratulations" to multiple requests for more information on the changes I have made in my diet and lifestyle. Cancer patients frequently ask of both their health care practitioner and themselves, "What else can I be doing to help fight my cancer, reduce my risks of a recurrence, or even keep a new cancer from developing?". Almost everyone who called asked me to write a book giving more information about my experiences, the changes I have made in my diet and lifestyle in order to address these important questions, and my resources.

A breast cancer survivor calling from New Jersey told me **the unique combination of both my lengthy experience as a cancer patient and survivor in conjunction with my clinical training as a Registered Dietitian gave her confidence that I would not allow myself to be "steered wrong" about the choices I made for recovering from this latest cancer.** She accurately summarized my approach to recovery this time. I tried diligently to simultaneously wear both my "patient and clinician hats" as I explored which conventional cancer therapy was right for me along with which "alternative or complementary" therapies might supplement and enhance (not replace) the conventional treatments for my most recent cancer.

I wrote this book to give those people interested in an integrated and comprehensive approach for optimizing health after cancer a "jump start" onto that path. It is precisely what I wish my own cancer center could have had available to give me when I asked, "What else can I be doing?" It gives the details of my own path and journey. It is a concise guidebook, not an overwhelming, detailed travel log, nor is it a tightly scheduled itinerary on a tour bus. You can pick and choose the strategies that appeal to you when you are ready to incorporate them into your life.

I wish you the very best for both optimal health and healing after your cancer diagnosis. Thank you all for your prayers, best wishes, and confidence in me.

I was diagnosed with neuroblastoma, a childhood cancer, when I was 6 months old in 1950. It was treated successfully with surgery plus very large doses of radiation therapy, and I had a normal, healthy childhood. However, my parents, and later I, were extra vigilant regarding my subsequent health, always wondering if any additional health problems might develop secondary to the radiation therapy that cured me of my first cancer. I first had two "cancer scares" developing a thyroid tumor in 1962 and ovarian tumors in 1972, both of which, thankfully, were benign. In 1981, I sought out the advice of an oncologist regarding my concerns about the potential for still developing any subsequent cancer. As he discussed what was known and what wasn't known yet about breast cancer risk following radiation at a young age, I remember thinking that "breast cancer was for 'old' women - I didn't really need to worry about that yet." However, I did start doing monthly self breast exams which likely saved my life just 3 years later.

When I was 34 years old, I discovered a lump in my left breast, which had clearly not been there the month before. I had even had a breast exam by my physician 3 weeks earlier with no sign of a lump (and I remember commenting to him that I felt terrific!). Upon biopsy, the lump was determined to be malignant, an invasive intra-ductal carcinoma with indeterminate estrogen receptor status. Due to the large amount of radiation I received after my neuroblastoma diagnosis, a lumpectomy followed by radiation therapy was not an option for me. Therefore, I had a modified radical mastectomy with lymph node dissection, which showed one positive node. I underwent 6 cycles of chemotherapy (Cytoxan, Methotrexate, and 5-FU) and took the anti-estrogen drug Tamoxifen for one year. After that time period was over, I submerged my fears about what might still come and coped by adopting the simple belief that this was now all behind me. I jumped back into my life, which centered on my husband, Dick, raising my two sons, Eric, age 7 and Garrison, age 2, and developing my career.

My second breast cancer was first noticed as a suspicious area seen on my 10 year anniversary mammogram, and subsequently determined to be malignant after a biopsy. I was shocked and really angry this time - I couldn't believe it! My life was in full swing - I had no time slots open in my Franklin Planner for cancer again! And why was this still happening to me? I thought I had lived a very healthy lifestyle, and I also thought, "I'd paid my dues" by having cancer twice already. This was a brand new cancer, not a recurrence. Therefore, while it seemed surgery and chemotherapy had cured me of my first breast cancer, just choosing those two modalities of treatment were obviously not enough to keep a new cancer from developing in me. Besides, even though my new tumor was small (1.4 cm), this cancer was much more advanced than my first breast cancer, having 9 positive axillary lymph nodes and 1 positive deep intermammary lymph node found with a PET scan, putting me at very high risk for recurrence this time.

It was time to start looking at things in a new way. I never questioned that chemotherapy and surgery would play a role in my treatment with this second breast cancer. However, because of my apparent high risk factors from the radiation therapy and who knows what else, **I now knew I could no longer naively think that chemo and surgery alone were all I needed to do to keep this cancer from coming back or even another new one from developing.**

I was finally ready to turn around in order to both confront and embrace my cancer history. In addition, I knew that it was finally time for me to go beyond coping (which I had obviously done very well for 45 years!) to healing - physically, emotionally, and spiritually. Although I was choosing a mastectomy and chemotherapy (Adriamycin and Cytoxan) as the first line offense against my disease, I was determined to figure out what else I could do to enhance the long-term effectiveness of these treatments by identifying and changing various aspects of my lifestyle.

The challenge that I accepted for myself was to see if I could put together a "healing recipe", looking for the best ingredients that conventional oncology therapy had to offer and complementing it with additional therapies from the uncharted world of "alternative medicine" and as such, see if I could "tweak my fate".

I remember telling my husband after chemotherapy was completed that as hard as the previous six months had been, I knew that the next 6 months were going to be even more difficult. The process of doing a life review and determining what aspects to change that might offer some hope for reducing my cancer odds was daunting. It was not a quick process, nor an easy one. I started by coming home from my last chemotherapy session thinking "Now what?" and feeling very alone, lost and abandoned. (Feeling abandoned by the medical system of which professionally I was a part was doubly difficult.) As I left my last chemo session, no one even told me good-bye or good luck. More importantly, I wish that someone would have handed me a little "map" or a guidebook for the options I had for the multiple lifestyle changes that could be considered for their potential of both reducing my risks of recurrence and facilitating healing. I hope this book serves as that "map" or guidebook.

I'm fully aware and accept that there are "no guarantees" for cancer recovery. Cancer is a disease that has baffled the best scientists, physicians, and healers over the ages, but I don't believe anyone will dispute there are lifestyle changes that can be done to tip the scales in a person's favor for both fighting the disease and achieving the optimal health possible. All the research studies aren't done, many of them haven't even been started yet, however, I didn't have time to wait for all the answers to be defined to the complete satisfaction of the scientific community before I made changes.

Therefore, I have tried to determine what is known, what's not, what's controversial, what's harmless to try, what's least expensive, what offers real hope compared to hype or even potential harm, and subsequently developed a "healing recipe" for myself. It is my belief that no one ingredient has been the "magic bullet" responsible for my healing. I also believe true healing does not have to be a "cure" and is only possible through a holistic, multi-faceted approach providing for my physical, emotional, mental, and spiritual needs. In addition, I don't believe there is only one right answer. Chi Kung and soy shakes might be right for me, but yoga and various teas right for you.

I share with you my two favorite quotations:

> ❆ "I encourage my patients to have faith in God
> but not to expect Him (Her) to do all the work."
> - Dr. Bernie Siegel, *Love, Medicine, and Miracles*

> ❆ "When the dog is chasing you, turn around and whistle for it."
> - Henry David Thoreau

Both of them have been very inspirational to me as I have worked at recovering and healing after my latest cancer.

I am now four years past my most recent diagnosis and still considered cancer-free. It is amazing to me how much I have changed during this time. I have made many major lifestyle changes already, but I am still working on others. While I wouldn't wish cancer on anyone, I do know that I have a sense of accomplishment, satisfaction, and contentment with my life right now that wouldn't be there without my latest cancer experience. It is my hope that some aspect of this book will be resonate with you and be helpful as you begin your journey toward recovery and healing after cancer.

Why did I think I needed to change my diet? Wasn't I, as a dietitian, eating healthy before? Yes, I was. I had cut back to eating bratwurst only once each year, ate my "5-A-Day", cut my overall fat intake to 30% years ago, ate double cheese pizza and high fat yummy ice cream only "in moderation" - all the "right things" according to published guidelines to reduce cancer risk. Maybe eating as healthfully as I had been kept me from getting my two breast cancers sooner, maybe even helped keep me alive after my first one. However, if I, as a dietitian, believed at all that "we are what we eat", I felt compelled after my second breast cancer to accept the challenge of changing my food intake to create a biochemical environment in my body that was potentially less conducive and/or more protective against cancer. *I wanted everything I put in my mouth to truly help maximize my potential for long-term survival from cancer.*

Research to understand the "optimal" diet to treat cancer, prevent cancer or a recurrence is still on-going and evolving. Many questions are still unanswered, particularly regarding how, when, what type, and amounts of dietary fats contribute to the development of cancer. The same questions are still not fully understood regarding the role soy might have in preventing cancer. However, it is reassuring to know there are over 200 studies reported in the scientific literature showing diets high in fruits and vegetables reduce the risk of many types of cancer. In fact, research is "mushrooming" in the new area of phytochemicals (non-nutrient components of plants) and the role of these compounds from our food in the prevention and treatment of cancer.

The American Cancer Society, The National Cancer Institute, and The American Institute for Cancer Research have published dietary guidelines based on multiple research studies. Knowing there are "no guarantees", using these guidelines and other information in the scientific literature, I have created my own nutrition "action plan" to help minimize my risk of both recurrent breast cancer and even a potential brand new type of cancer.

My own professional organizations might say I've unnecessarily taken my diet to a point that is not yet scientifically supported. However, they would also say that my diet is nutritionally adequate, healthy, and not dangerous in any way. In fact, it was because my risk of recurrence was so high (and there are still so many "loose ends" with the entire nutrition and cancer connection) that I created this diet for myself in order to address many of those still unanswered questions. I needed to personally draw a line in the sand on many controversial questions such as how much and what types of fat to include in my diet, how many and which types of fruits and vegetables to eat, organic vs. non-organic foods, how much soy (if any) to include. The questions go on and on.

I have worked hard over the past 3+ years, first by reading extensively in the scientific nutritional literature to more clearly understand what was known, what was not, and what is considered controversial in the field of cancer and nutrition. I've spoken personally with many researchers to both make sure I was understanding their research and to see what their thoughts were regarding the diet plan I was developing for myself.

In addition, I worked hard in my own kitchen to see if this ultra-healthy diet was indeed "doable". Could a dietitian who had only tasted soy milk at a conference and never incorporated tofu into her family's diet do more than "talk the talk"? Could I actually "walk the walk"? I have done it, and you can, too. It is workable, tasty, and enjoyable, and, I have done it with a minimum of stress or obsession.

My family was a good sport about all my changes and tried everything for the first 6-9 months or so. At some point though, they politely put their collective foot down and said, "No more beans every night or tofu hot dogs!" So I began figuring out how to do this for me without cooking two complete meals (more time, more stress), and I have included some of my tips for that, too.

I had many difficulties tolerating my chemotherapy during which time I admittedly ate "whatever I could". I did not fully implement this entire new nutrition plan until after I completed my chemo and was starting to regain my strength, lose my "chemo brain", and have my taste sensations begin to normalize. For those of you with a better tolerance to your chemo, I would strongly suggest implementing these changes as soon after your diagnosis as possible. In fact, I have heard from hundreds of people who have already bought this book that making these changes has been easier than they thought and also beneficial. Many, many people have called me or written to say my shake recipe "got them through chemo" and also helped them with full recovery by "energizing" them ! So wherever you are in your cancer journey, it's never to early to start with changes, but it's not too late either. Every change you make is one step toward both improving your chances for long-term survival from cancer and your quality of life.

Don't feel overwhelmed though! It took me almost a year after I completed my chemotherapy to fully implement this plan for myself and still be able to feed my family, too! You'll be able to do it faster because I was researching at the same time. So, start by making a goal of experimenting and changing one component per month in your diet. Start by changing what seems easiest to you. Maybe that will be making my shake every day. Next you might try to consistently incorporate 9+ servings of fruits and veggies into your daily diet. *Every little change is potentially helpful, and any change is better than none.* You can do it!

The following information consists of general guidelines. You may have a medical condition for which additional modification of these guidelines would be appropriate. Please discuss any planned changes with your health care professionals. Every cancer center should have a Registered Dietitian (RD) on its staff available to assess your nutritional requirements and make specific suggestions. If a dietitian is not available at your cancer center, or the staffing is inadequate, advocate for increased accessibility to an RD so nutrition services can be available in both a pro-active and in-depth manner. Don't wait until you have lost or gained a significant amount of weight to see a dietitian for information to help you.

The following components of my diet plan are listed in order of importance to me personally, and also, as I best understand the strength of the scientific evidence for their role in the nutrition and cancer connection.

Nutritional Components

- Prepare and eat all meals in a loving, caring manner. The fast food era of our life is a thing of the past. This has required a major life-style change to which I am committed. I can't tell you how to do this for your own family, but it was *the* most important thing for me. We eat sit-down meals without the TV or dashing somewhere almost every night of the week. I do think of the time I spend fixing meals everyday as a necessary "ingredient" in my total healing "recipe".

- Achieve and maintain a healthy weight for height. Regular exercise is very important both to achieve a healthy weight and in its own right for maximizing the function of our immune system. When I really forced myself to examine how frequently I exercised prior to this latest cancer, I had to admit I exercised "whenever I could". I was not faithful. I now regularly walk 2-3 miles 5-7 days/week, striving for a minimum of 4 hours/week of vigorous exercise.

- Eliminate/reduce alcohol intake. This was not hard for me to change. When I do occasionally have a drink, I choose a red wine or a dark beer, both of which have higher phytochemical contents than white wine or regular beer.

[5]

🍎 Increase fiber to 25-30 gm/day. The average American intake is 10-12 gm/day, and I was *not* above average before. Wow, was that hard to admit!
- 6 servings/day of whole grain foods (>6 if higher calories needed)
- 1-2 servings/day of legumes
- 5-9+ servings/day of fruits and vegetables, at least 3 different colors each day, consider using organic produce when available (See additional information in Appendix)

A fiber intake of this amount is easy to achieve when your diet is based on fruits, vegetables and whole grains. I now have a personal goal of a *minimum* of 9 servings of fruits and vegetables each day. I aim for 3 servings at each meal plus snacks of fruits or vegetables each day. The darkest colored fruits and vegetables have the highest content of phytochemicals. Toss out your iceberg lettuce and use spinach, kale, romaine, leaf lettuce, or other greens instead.

You may need to increase fiber gradually to minimize GI distress. Use of a product like Beano® from your drug store will help cut down gas production from legumes until your body adapts to a regular intake. I always have some legumes cooked and in the refrig or freezer to use. I also use a lot of canned cooked beans since they are so fast and easy to keep on the pantry shelf.

🍎 Reduce fat in your diet to approximately 20% of your caloric intake.
- 16-18% fat in our diet is the minimum amount required in order to maximize the absorption of the fat-soluble (cancer-fighting) phytochemicals. The very low fat diets (10% or less) for reversing heart disease are likely too low in fat to maximize their cancer reduction potential. This is where identifying your medical and nutritional priorities is important and individualizing a diet plan can best be done with the guidance of a Registered Dietitian.

- Consume a small amount of fat with between meal fruit and vegetable snacks to ensure maximum absorption of the phytochemicals. Most of the phytochemicals are fat-soluble like beta-carotene and Vitamin A and need some fat eaten with them to get the highest quantity possible absorbed and into the blood stream so they can do their cancer-fighting action in your body's cells. I will eat a small amount of soynut butter (like peanut butter), soy nuts (easy to carry in my purse and/or brief case), nuts, pine nuts, or hummus along with my between meal fruit and veggie snacks.

- I will, at the present time, avoid the new synthetic fat substitute that impairs absorption of both fat-soluble vitamins and phytochemicals as it mixes with food in our GI tract. The product is being fortified with the fat-soluble vitamins to minimize this effect for vitamins A, D, E, and K. No phytochemicals are currently being added to this product. Since there are hundreds, if not thousands, of phytochemicals in our food that may be playing very important roles in preventing cancer and other degenerative diseases, I want all of them to be maximally absorbed into my body. I will be following the research on this product and phytochemicals very closely.

- Use only extra-virgin olive oil or canola oil in your regular cooking. Eliminate regular margarine, liquid corn oil and other vegetable/seed oils from regular use. Olive and canola oil are highest in the monounsaturated fats that may or may not confer protection against cancer, but do not appear to be potentially carcinogenic as the omega-6 fatty acids may be that are predominant in vegetable oils like corn oil. I still occasionally use a small amount of dark sesame oil for flavoring Asian recipes. Using my blender, I began combining butter and olive oil into a spread for fresh bread, but now there is at least one commercial product available with > 50% olive oil that fits this niche. Additionally, there are a few margarine products entering the market that are free of "trans-fatty acids", which are the hydrogenated, or partially-hardened, polyunsaturated fats that may also contribute to increased cancer risk.

❦ Reduced fats (cont.):
  • Example: for an intake of 1600-1800-2000 calories/day, a 20% fat diet would equal 36-40-44 grams of fat per day. You have to read food labels and be honest about serving sizes that you are eating. Have a dietitian help you figure your approximate caloric needs and resulting range of fat intake to consume.

❦ Buy only very lean meats and reduce portion size to 2-3 oz./meal (approximately the size of a deck of playing cards). Think of meats as an "accent" for the other food items on a plate instead of the "main attraction". Consider using meat/poultry grown without hormones or antibiotics. I have eliminated all meats and poultry from my diet. For my family, I have reduced the frequency and amounts of meats I serve them, and I also buy organically-raised meats when available.

❦ If you can tolerate dairy products, use only reduced-fat (not no-fat) dairy products, consuming 1-3 servings/day. Dairy fat has the highest concentration of a molecule called "conjugated linoleic acid" or "CLA" for short, which has anti-cancer activity and may be present in higher concentration in organic milk products. Consider using dairy products from non-BST (growth hormone) treated cows as they contain lower levels of a molecule called Insulin-like Growth Factor (IGF-1). Higher blood levels of IGF-1 have been associated with several types of cancer. Much more research needs to be completed to clarify the relationship between IGF-1 and cancer, but I consider this a "loose end" and prefer to eliminate this possible risk factor from my diet. I now use only organic dairy products from non-BST treated cows for myself. Some products I can buy in my regular grocery store, but others I get at a health food store. My family has increased the frequency of consumption of these products too, but they do not eat them exclusively. When we go out for pizza, I order mine with extra vegetables and no cheese. When we make pizza at home, I use soy cheese.

❦ Consume soy products 1-3 servings/day. Soybeans have many anti-carcinogenic compounds, some of which (the phytoestrogen genistein) are unique to soybeans. We do not yet know the exact amount of soy in our diet to consume for a protective or therapeutic benefit. We also don't know which cancers may be prevented by soy or benefit from soy consumption as part of treatment, or even if soy will be able to confer any protection or benefits if one continues to eat a high fat diet low in plant foods. However current research shows that even as little as one serving each day may offer some advantage to reducing your cancer risk. Similar to a traditional Japanese diet, I consume 1-3 servings of soy foods daily, primarily from soymilk, tofu, tempeh, soybeans, soynut butter, and miso. Not all soy foods, such as some "veggie burgers", currently have all of the important cancer fighting compounds due to the processing of the soy protein. Products made from "isolated" soy protein will contain more of the phytoestrogens (also called isoflavones) than products made with "concentrated" soy protein. Be sure to read food labels. Some companies are even starting to add the isoflavone content of their product on the labels.

I currently advise my clients to focus on introducing soy foods, rather than supplements, into their diet in order to take advantage of the multiple anti-carcinogenic properties that whole soy foods potentially have to offer. *Don't go overboard though*. Eating a pound of tofu every day may be potentially harmful due to large amount of phytoestrogens. Currently, confusion and controversy surround the inclusion of soy products for those people with cancers that are hormone-responsive. An example would be a woman with ER+, post-menopausal breast cancer, being treated with the anti-estrogen drug Tamoxifen. (I myself fit this profile.) Do the phytoestrogens in soy "fuel" cancer growth? Do they compete with and make the Tamoxifen less effective? Do they possibly even enhance Tamoxifen's benefits? Are they neutral or even beneficial for reducing cancer risk in their own right? I will be following the research in this area very closely. We don't know all the answers yet, however, I am professionally "comfortable" consuming 1-3 servings of soy on a daily basis and have been doing this for the past 3+ years without a recurrence.

- Consume cold water fish 2-3x/week (approx. 1 pound/week). Salmon, mackerel, white tuna, sardines, bluefish, ocean trout, and herring are all high in the omega-3 fatty acids that may help fight cancer. Of these, I only like salmon and tuna and make an effort to eat approximately 1# total each week. Almost all restaurants have salmon on the menu now which makes it easier to go out to eat. Fortunately my whole family loves seafood, so 2 meals each week are easy to fix for all of us to eat the same food together.

- Limit grilled, broiled, "blackened" meats and fish to special occasions only. This type of cooking, unfortunately, produces carcinogens. Steamed, microwaved, baked, boiled, poached, or stewed food preparation is healthier. (Grilling veggies does not produce the same carcinogens.) Marinating meats prior to grilling does greatly reduce the carcinogens produced.

- Liberally make use of various herbs and spices in your cooking for both enhancing flavor with low fat foods and increasing your intake of phytochemicals that may have a role in fighting cancer. Use a wide variety. (See page 27 for a list of culinary herbs with anti-cancer activity.)

- Flax seeds, ground seed meal, and flax seed oil are a plant source of an omega-3 fatty acid that may be valuable to help fight cancer. In addition, flax seeds, but not the oil, are the most concentrated plant source of a phytochemical, lignan, that bacteria in our large bowel convert to a molecule with "anti-estrogen" properties which may be useful in preventing or treating tumors that are estrogen responsive. I use 1-2 Tbsp. of ground flax meal/day. The optimal amount to include in our diets to prevent or treat cancer, and which cancers, is the subject of much current research.

What Counts as a Serving Size?

- Meats :
  - 2-3 ounces of cooked lean meat, poultry or fish

- Dairy Foods and Eggs:
  - 1 cup milk or yogurt
  - 2 ounces processed cheese
  - 1-1/2 oz. natural cheese
  - 1 egg

- Grains:
  - 1 slice of bread, 1/2 bagel, 1 dinner roll
  - 1/2 cup cooked cereal, rice or pasta
  - 1 ounce ready to eat cereal

- Beans and Nuts:
  - 1/2 cup cooked dry beans
  - 1/3 cup nuts
  - 2 Tbsp. peanut butter

- Fruit:
  - 1 medium apple, banana or orange
  - 1/2 cup chopped, cooked, or canned fruit
  - 3/4 cup fruit juice
  - 1/4 cup dried fruit

- Vegetables:
  - 1 cup raw leafy vegetables
  - 1/2 cup other cooked or raw vegetables, chopped
  - 3/4 cup vegetable juice

- Soy products:
  - 1 cup soy milk
  - 1/2 cup tempeh
  - 1/2 cup rehydrated textured vegetable protein (TVP)
  - 1/2 cup (4 oz.) tofu
  - 2 tablespoons soy nuts
  - 1/4 cup soy butter

How to Achieve 9+ Servings/Day of Fruits and Vegetables without Chomping Carrots All Day Long!

As a dietitian, I knew I was eating my "5-A-Day" quite consistently. I made a new goal to consume a minimum of 9 servings daily to better assist my body's biochemistry with the cancer-fighting phytochemicals. I wanted to do that by eating whole foods but, I had trouble imagining how I would eat more! I've found it's actually not that hard to do, but it does take thought and planning. It doesn't happen by accident. Here are some helpful suggestions:

- My soy shake recipes on pages 12 and 13 each contain 3 servings of fruit and veggies. That is my breakfast each morning. I can't drink it all right away, so what I don't finish at breakfast, I put into an insulated coffee mug with a lid and a straw and drink over the next hour or so.
- Fresh or dried fruit for between meal snacks. I keep dried fruit in a "ziploc" bag inside my briefcase. I also will throw in an apple or banana, too.
- Drink 100% juices between meals. I have given up pop. I like a new product, a combined 100% fruit and vegetable juice in a juicebox, that is easy to carry with me.
- Make up large amounts of tossed salad with lots of extra veggies cut up in them so you are getting a variety. Also, that way you've got a salad ready for tomorrow's lunch or supper already. I use the new vegetable storage plastic bags to help keep all the veggies fresh.
- Add fruit to salads like apples, mandarin oranges, dried cranberries or cherries.
- Mix fruit with plain yogurt for a snack.
- Cut up an assortment of veggies to be readily available for snacks. I often have red pepper strips with hummus for an afternoon snack.
- Add extra vegetables to soups, either homemade or canned.
- Decrease or even eliminate the meat and cheese in a sandwich and increase the veggies - extra lettuce, tomato, alfalfa sprouts, pepper strips, avocado.
- Buy tabouli already made in the deli section of your grocery store for a quick and easy source of numerous phytochemicals.
- Load up with lots of raw veggies at the salad bar, like dark lettuce and spinach - not iceberg.
- Make kebobs for the grill that are veggies and fruit with zucchini, yellow squash, onion, mushrooms, cherry tomatoes, sweet peppers, eggplant, pineapple wedges, peach slices, etc.
- Thawed frozen fruit on top of angel food cake makes a nice dessert.
- Keep a small box of raisins in your desk at work, briefcase, or the car.
- Make low fat quiche with veggies. I use up left-over veggies this way.
- Keep plenty of salsa on hand as a dip for veggies or low-fat chips.
- Try a new fruit or veggie each week. Grocery stores often have dietitians working for them now to help you with cooking ideas. At the very least, the stores will have recipe cards to guide you with something new.
- Buy small snack-packs of canned fruit to take for lunch.
- Mix last night's left over veggies into tonight's salad.
- When you're baking anything, throw into the oven some potatoes, sweet potatoes, and winter squash for that day or later in the week to reheat in the microwave when you have less time.
- Have a baked potato and juice at a fast food restaurant. Top the potato with salsa.
- Look for already peeled, sliced, or even shredded fruits and/or vegetables at the grocery store for ultimate convenience.
- Put extra veggies into spaghetti sauce. Shredded carrots are nice.
- We serve stir-fried veggies once every week. We vary the meat and veggie (I use tofu, tempeh, or simply some beans with mine).
- Make a veggie pizza with lots of broccoli, mushrooms, peppers, artichoke hearts, onions, dried tomatoes.
- Make reduced-fat fruit desserts like baked apples, crisps, and cobblers.

Even my family eats 6-9 servings/day of fruits and vegetables now. Be creative and give it a try. You'll be surprised. It's easier than you think!

Sample Menu:

- **Breakfast**
  My shake. One day I might use mangos and raspberries for the fruit ingredients and another day I might use only blueberries. Experiment. Sometimes I even use left-over sweet potatoes instead of the carrots. I use a brand of soy milk that is highest in protein and fortified with calcium. (See my grocery list in the Appendix.)

- **Morning Snack**
  3/4 cup of pink grapefruit juice (higher in phytochemicals than plain)
  4-5 low-fat crackers

- **Lunch**
  Dehydrated bean soup in one of those cardboard containers (look for one that is highest in protein and fiber and lowest in sodium) or homemade soup, left-over veggie-type casserole
  Whole-grain bagel
  1/2 pink grapefruit
  1/2 sweet red pepper cut into strips with some hummus for dip
  1 8-oz. carton fruit/veggie juice

- **Afternoon snack**
  5-6 dried apricots
  4-5 almonds

- **Supper**
  I might cook my family baked chicken with crispy bread crumbs according to a Jane Brody recipe. For myself, I would bake a couple slices of extra-firm tofu coated with the bread crumb mixture, too, right along with the chicken.
  1 cup instant brown rice
  1 cup steamed fresh or frozen broccoli
  1 cup tossed salad with romaine lettuce, kale, and other veggies
  1 cup 1% milk
  I use 1-2 teaspoons of olive oil and a flavored vinegar for dressing on my salad. I also would put about 1 teaspoon of the butter/olive oil spread on my broccoli for extra flavor and also to get the fat amount up to 20% of the diet.

- **PM Snack**
  8 oz. low-fat yogurt
  1/2 apple with 1 teaspoon soy butter
  Decaffeinated tea of various kinds

This is just one sample menu. It contains approximately 2000 calories, 45 gm fat (20%), 12 servings of fruits and vegetables. 5-6 servings of whole grains (I count the fiber I get from the wheat bran and wheat germ in the shake, too), 2-3 servings of soy, 1 serving of legumes, 2 dairy products, plenty of high quality protein from the dairy, legumes, and soy products, and overall, a very balanced and healthful diet.

Additional Tips for Integrating this Diet with a Family

- It's only the entree that I have to think about. Everything else is the same.
- Fortunately, my family loves seafood of any kind, so we regularly have two seafood meals each week.
- We have "stir-fry" once each week, always varying the vegetables and the meats. It's easy to make this both with and without added meat. For myself, I might add tofu, tempeh, seitan (a wheat gluten product), or beans.
- The veggie burgers come in handy when my family wants burgers. I would even make one for myself if they are having something like pork chops.

- There are "meat substitutes" for bacon, sausage, hot dogs, chicken nuggets, etc. I use those whenever needed as a substitute for the real thing for me.
- Tacos, burritos, fajitas are all easy. I can make mine with just beans at the same time I'm making theirs.
- I use the frozen textured vegetable protein that looks and cooks just like cooked ground hamburger for spaghetti sauce, chili, sloppy joes, etc.
- If I'm making a recipe that has a sauce of any kind, I just substitute tofu for the meat, like in chicken cacciatorie, in a separate pan or baking dish for me.
- If we order delivery pizza, I have enough time to make my own using whole wheat pizza crust or pita bread, tomato sauce, fresh veggies, and tofu mozzarella cheese.

Sources for Recipes that I've Used and Loved

Jane Brody's Good Food Book, W.W. Norton and Co., 1985.
Jane Brody's Good Food Gourmet, Bantam Publishers, 1990.
Jane Brody's Good Seafood Book, Balantine Publishers, 1994.
All of Jane Brody's cookbooks emphasize low fat eating, the significant reduction of the amount of meats eaten while increasing consumption of whole grains, fruits, and vegetables. These are terrific cookbooks to start with if you're not ready to be 100% vegetarian yet.

High Fit - Low Fat Vegetarian, E.R. Burt, I.A.C.P., K.B. Goldberg, M.S., R.D., K.S. Rhodes, Ph.D., R.D., University of Michigan Medical Center, Ann Arbor, MI, 1996. Wonderful recipes.

The Vegetarian Way: Total Health for You and Your Family, M. Messina, Ph.D. and V. Messina, MPH, RD, Crown Trade Paperbacks, New York, 1996. Very good information about vegetarian diets along with recipes.

The Simple Soybean and Your Health, M. Messina, Ph.D., V. Messina, R.D., and K. Setchell, Ph.D., Avery Publishing Group, Garden City Park, NY, 1994. A great overview of the potential health benefits of including soybeans in a diet with several good recipes for getting started.

Simply Soy: A Variety of Choices, K. Rhodes, Ph.D., R.D. and C. Sullivan, M.A. R.D., The Michigan Soybean Promotion Committee, P.O. Box 287, Frankenmuth, MI 48734, call (517) 652-3294. 1997. This entire booklet is available on the Internet at: http://soyfoods.com/SimplySoy

Life Tastes Better than Steak Cookbook, Gerry Krag, M.A., R.D. and Marie Zimolzak, D.T.R, Avery Color Studios, Marquette, MI, 1996. Great vegetarian recipes and what a profound title!

Simple, Lowfat and Vegetarian: Unbelievably Easy Ways to Reduce the Fat in Your Meals!, Suzanne Havala, M.S. R.D., Vegetarian Resource Group, P.O. Box 1463, Baltimore, MD, 1994. This is more than just recipes - this is a book about how to eat this way in real life (from restaurants to amusement parks!).

Meatless Meals for Working People: Quick and Easy Vegetarian Recipes, D. Wasserman and C. Stahler, The Vegetarian Resource Group, P.O. Box 1463, Baltimore, MD, 1996.

Lickety-Split Meals for Health Conscious People on the Go!, Zonya Foco, RD, 1-888-884-LEAN. Great recipes, all of which have tips for making them meatless. I love the clever design of this book. It stands up on my kitchen counter with the recipe easy to read.

Vegetarian Cooking for Healthy Living, M. Ter Meer, BS, and J. Galeana, MS, RD. Great recipes, easy to follow with common ingredients. 1-800-322-5679.

I developed these shake recipes to provide beneficial phytochemicals (non-nutrient plant molecules) that are now thought to have multiple cancer-fighting activities. The shakes are all easy to prepare, consume, and digest. There are more than 1000 phytochemicals in our foods from fruits, vegetables, whole grains, soy foods and other legumes. **I drink one entire shake for breakfast daily.** I consider it the centerpiece of my diet plan. It could also be consumed between meals. *Many* people have called or written me to say how tasty the shakes are and additionally, how helpful they have been with "getting through chemo" and "energizing" them. Drink to your health and enjoy!

The contents of a full recipe contain 3 servings from the fruit and vegetable groups, approximately 1-1/2 servings of soy, 40-60% of your daily calcium requirement, 33-40% of your daily fiber requirement, and a healthy dose of phytochemicals too numerous to count!

Recipe #1 is completely lactose free, which is beneficial for those people that are lactose intolerant either prior to or temporarily during cancer therapy. Recipes #2-4 are low in lactose and also, contain active bacterial cultures from the yogurt, which help maintain healthy, normal intestinal flora and may also help reduce cancer.

❦ RECIPE #1

2-1/2 oz. soft tofu (cut a 1 lb. block of tofu into 6 pieces)
6-8 baby carrots or one large carrot
3/4 cup fresh or frozen unsweetened fruit
1 Tbsp. wheat bran
1 Tbsp. wheat germ
1 Tbsp. whole flax seed or ground flax seed meal
3/4 cup calcium fortified soy milk
3/4 cup calcium-fortified orange juice

Put ingredients into a blender. Start blender on a lower speed, then increase to high for 1-3 minutes to fully blend ingredients (variable time depending on blender's motor strength).

Makes about 3 cups. Approximate nutritional content:

Calories	450 kcal	Protein	25 gm	Fat	10 gm
Fiber	14 gm	Calcium	475 mg		

❦ RECIPE #2

6-8 baby carrots or one large carrot
3/4 cup fresh or frozen unsweetened fruit
3 Tbsp. frozen juice concentrate (not diluted)
2-1/2 oz. tofu (cut a 1 lb. block of tofu into 6 pieces)
1 cup calcium fortified soy milk
1 cup low-fat plain yogurt
1 Tbsp. wheat germ
1 Tbsp. wheat bran
1 Tbsp. whole flax seeds or ground flax seed meal

Makes about 3-1/2 cups. Approximate nutritional content:

Calories	580 kcal	Protein	38 gm	Fat	11 gm
Fiber	14 gm	Calcium	725 mg		

♣ RECIPE #3
8 oz. (1 cup) calcium fortified soy milk
8 oz. (1 cup) vanilla low-fat yogurt
6-8 baby carrots or one large carrot
1/2 cup fresh fruit (mango is nice)
3/4 cup frozen fruit (raspberries make a pretty shake)
1 Tbsp. wheat germ
1 Tbsp. wheat bran
1 Tbsp. whole flax seeds or ground flax meal
2-1/2 oz. tofu (cut a 1 lb. block of tofu into 6 pieces)

Makes about 3-1/2 cups. Approximate nutritional content:

Calories	658 kcal	Protein	35 gm	Fat	12 gm
Fiber	12 gm	Calcium	690 mg		

♣ RECIPE #4
3/4 cup calcium-fortified orange juice
8 oz. (1 cup) low-fat plain yogurt
4 oz. tofu (cut a 1 lb. block of tofu into 4 equal pieces)
6-8 baby carrots or 1 large carrot
3/4 cup frozen unsweetened fruit
1 Tbsp. wheat germ
1 Tbsp. wheat bran
1 Tbsp. whole flax seeds or ground meal

Makes about 3 cups. Approximate nutritional content:

Calories	520 kcal	Protein	31 gm	Fat	9 gm
Fiber	12 gm	Calcium	750 mg		

Additional Helpful Hints:
- ♣ Look for tofu in the produce section of the grocery store. It should be kept cool.
- ♣ Change the tofu water daily.
- ♣ **If you are severely immune-suppressed during or after your cancer therapy, you must minimize your risk of food-born illness. Ask your cancer center for a copy of their guidelines of foods to avoid.**
- ♣ I maximize my calcium intake (to help treat my osteoporosis) by using a brand of tofu that is higher in calcium (made with calcium sulfate or gypsum, not nigari), and calcium-fortified orange juice and soy milk.
- ♣ Buying both wheat bran and wheat germ in bulk at a health food store is much cheaper.
- ♣ Choose a brand of soy milk that is highest in protein and calcium.
- ♣ If an even less sweet shake is more appealing (especially while you are on chemo), add frozen cranberries as part of the fruit.
- ♣ Buy whole flax seeds at a health food store. To make your own flax meal, grind about 1/2 cup in a blender for a few seconds, then store both seeds and the ground meal in the freezer.
- ♣ Buy yogurt that contains active, live bacterial cultures.
- ♣ If you have mouth sores during cancer therapy, do not choose fruits that contain tiny seeds (such as blackberries) which can be irritating. Choose fruit or fruit juice that is non-acidic. Some cancer patients say that yogurt and buttermilk are both soothing and speed healing of mouth sores. Buttermilk could be substituted for yogurt in any of the shakes.
- ♣ Start with small amounts of wheat germ, bran, and flax. Then gradually increase to the full amount. Be sure to drink lots of non-caffeinated fluids as you increase your fiber intake.

There are approximately 1500 deaths from cancer daily in the U.S. (~ 1 death each *minute*, or the same as the Titanic sinking *every* day!). However, I prefer to concentrate and visualize myself in the group of cancer survivors, of which there are now approximately 10 million in the U.S. today, up from 6 million in 1990. Approximately 5 million of these survivors are now at least 5 years "out" from their diagnosis. Additionally, there are currently about 2.6 million breast cancer survivors. You are not alone, but instead are a member of quite a large "club"!

I would like to share the following quotations with you. They have been very meaningful to me as I have recovered from my latest cancer.

- "Survivorship, quite simply, begins when you are told you have cancer and continues for the rest of your life." Fitzhugh Mullan, M.D. (founder of the National Coalition of Cancer Survivorship)
- "Cancer survivorship is dynamic as opposed to static; it is not just about long-term survival. It goes beyond the disease and the response - or lack of response - to treatment. Rather survivorship permeates every aspect of your life after diagnosis." Susan Leigh, RN, BSN (survivor of 3 different cancers)
- "Successful survivorship does not need to equate to 'cure'. Healing is possible even when a cure is not." Michael Lerner, Ph.D. (founder of Commonweal, a cancer retreat center in California, and author, *Choices in Healing*)
- "It is necessary to hope...for hope itself is happiness." Samuel Johnson
- "Hope is the last to die." Russian Proverb

♣ CHARACTERISTICS AND SKILLS OF SURVIVORS ♣

I have been amazed to discover such an instant and deep bond with all of the cancer survivors who have called me, a total stranger, in response to the newspaper articles written about my life. As I talked to you and also thought about all the people I've known who have had cancer, I compiled a list of characteristics and skills that you all have demonstrated. I believe they are essential in order to maximize our chances of long-term survival, a sense of well-being, and true healing. Not everyone has perfected all of these characteristics and skills, but they are worth working on.

- Characteristics of Cancer Survivors:

Flexible	Resilient	Persistent
Forgiving	Hopeful	Pro-active
Out-spoken	Self-reliant	Sense of humor
Resourceful	Information seeker	Problem solver
Communicator	Negotiator	

  Self advocate, indeed a full partner, in your medical care
  Desire and have the ability to move forward in life
  Desire to evolve beyond "just surviving" to "thriving"
  Living life both joyfully and creatively

I have also observed in some of you, and personally experienced myself, both denial and anger with our cancer diagnoses and all the resultant problems that must now be addressed. My own personal belief is that both of these reactions are appropriate and should not be suppressed. They are both very effective coping tools and can serve a person well for a time. However, I believe for true *healing* to occur, a person must not get stuck in either of these two modes but must work to move beyond them in order to truly heal at all levels, physically, emotionally, mentally, and spiritually.

♣ MY "DECISION TREE" FOR EVALUATING ♣
AND IMPLEMENTING ANY ALTERNATIVE THERAPY

When I have worked at hospitals in the past, patients would occasionally bring in a large number of various dietary supplements that they wished to continue taking while hospitalized. That was my only exposure and source of information about the entire world of "alternative medicine" at that time. To step into that world made me more than a little uneasy, however, since I had decided to make significant changes to my diet, I was now very curious about what else was "out there" that offered promise to help reduce my risk for cancer recurrence.

My initial goal was to enhance my immune system to its maximum potential in order to help reduce my chances for cancer returning. During the 10+ years between my two breast cancers, my white blood cell counts never reached the normal range of 4000-10,000. Mine were always 2000-2500 and occasionally even lower. The explanation given to me was these low counts were to be expected with the amount of damage my bone marrow had sustained from both the radiation treatments that cured me of my childhood cancer and the chemotherapy that helped cure me of my first breast cancer. As a clinical scientist, I had always accepted that explanation as a reasonable consequence of past successes. However, after my third cancer, the patient part of my brain took over, and I no longer felt I could afford to accept that limitation as a "given". I was ready to try multiple means to augment my immune system - direct changes by altering my diet and introducing some herbs and vitamins, and indirect changes by some mind-body-spirit connection techniques.

I read extensively for the first year while I was making the changes in my diet. It would have been too overwhelming for me to change everything at once. Besides, I wanted to try to sort out what might offer some real hope.

As I read, I developed goals I wanted to achieve along with this thought process for myself to evaluate which strategies might be helpful for me. You may also think of other important questions to ask. In addition, these questions could also be applied to conventional therapies.
- Is there scientific evidence that this therapy will reduce/eliminate breast tumors of my type and stage (or "fill in the blank") in humans? What is the strength of the evidence? How does it work?
- Is there any evidence that this therapy may be potentially harmful for me?
- Is there evidence that this supplement or technique is harmless, or at the very best may increase my quality of life?
- Instead of "supplementation", is there a way to obtain the same (or better) result from food sources?
- How much money was I able and *willing* to spend not reimbursed by medical insurance?
- Does this therapy feel "right" in my heart/gut? Does this therapy "speak" to me? This question is important. It has allowed me to proceed with a therapy before having all the other questions answered to the satisfaction of my "left brain".
- Who should I choose as a practitioner/therapist/healer? What are their qualifications and my comfort level with them?
- Time considerations - "natural healing" takes time and effort - was I willing to invest that time and work for healing?
- Discuss this therapy with your oncologist or primary care physician. They may have some valid concerns regarding your particular medical condition. Become a full and equal partner on your medical team.

I cannot emphasize enough the importance of discussing all available therapeutic options, both conventional and complementary, with your physicians. Even if your physician never asks if you are interested and/or are already incorporating some complementary strategies into your cancer action plan, it is your responsibility to inform him/her. Speaking for myself, that takes courage! I found the courage because I have the *conviction* that these additional therapies are as important to my healing as the conventional therapies, and I wanted my physician to know that.

The following list is my current individual regimen for enhancing my body's anti-oxidant and immune systems. Does every cancer patient need these supplements or perhaps different ones or amounts? I don't know the full answer to that, and I don't believe anyone else does either. However, it now seemed apparent to me that a person like myself, with a tendency for developing cancer, needed something more than what I was getting from my previously healthy diet alone if I stood a chance to keep cancer from returning again. (I want to emphasize though that I think of these supplements as just that - "supplements" to help my ultra-healthy diet for optimal health, not "magic bullets" expected to compensate for an unhealthy diet and lifestyle.)

There is much controversy surrounding the pros and cons of taking anti-oxidants while also receiving chemo or radiation. So little is known at this time regarding the potential for large doses of antioxidants to perhaps protect cancer cells during chemo or radiation therapy, or even act as "pro-oxidants" causing more damage than protection of our healthy cells. It is highly likely to be very individualistic depending on tumor type and staging, drug mechanism of action, and many different individual biochemical characteristics. I hope much more research is done to determine the optimal supplementation beneficial for various cancers and each type of therapy.

I did not take any supplements at all while I was on chemo. I carefully eased into the world of supplements only after my chemo was finished. If you have a decreased nutritional intake during your cancer therapy, taking a one-a-day type of supplement providing 100% of the RDAs is appropriate. Additionally, ask to see the dietitian at your cancer center.

❦ Multi-vitamin and mineral supplement with approximately 100% RDA of everything - a brand with a lower amount of iron (10 mg or less per tablet)
❦ Vitamin C - 250 mg 2x/day
❦ Vitamin E - 200 IU - 1x/day - take with a meal/snack containing some fat to maximize absorption. Check expiration date of bottle. I use a natural (d-alpha) Vitamin E containing mixed tocopherols.
❦ Selenium - 100 mcg - from high selenium grown yeast 1x/day (100-200 mcg/day total is likely OK - be sure to see how much is in your multi-vitamin tablet. too)
❦ Calcium - 600-1200 mg/day - for my osteoporosis as is the Magnesium. I use calcium citrate.
❦ Magnesium - 250 mg/day - 1-2 tablets of MgOxide/day
❦ Echinacea root and herb - 400 mg capsule - an immune system enhancer. I take a "baby dose" of 1 capsule/day and increase to label recommendations at the first sign of a cold. I take it daily even though various references, but not all, advise taking only for 2-8 weeks and then waiting approximately 1 month before starting again.
❦ Astragalus membranaceus root (Chinese herb) - 470 mg capsules - again, an immune system enhancer - I take 1 capsule/day and only increase to label recs. at the first sign of a cold.
❦ Co-enzyme Q10 - 30-60 mg/day. An antioxidant. Optimal dosing to help prevent recurrence is not known yet. I based my dosage on what I am willing to spend/month.
❦ Teas - Astragalus, Ginseng, Green tea - 2-4 cups/day rotation

Although I am now officially a "pill popper", I still believe the overall health benefits I am receiving from my 9+ servings of fruits and vegetables and 1-3 servings of soy foods each day are even more important than the benefits of these supplements. **If I were forced to choose only one approach, I would put my money on maximizing my diet for the largest potential benefit.**

Additional information is included on pages 26-27 regarding how to choose brands of vitamins and herbs along with a few tips I give my clients about incorporating these supplements or any alternative/complementary therapy into their healing "recipe".

Besides changing my diet and adding some supplements, I have also included multiple new "ingredients" into my life to fully heal from this latest cancer - healing physically, emotionally, mentally, and spiritually. Going through this for the third time now gave me pause with reason to begin looking at everything in my life. I intuitively knew that I could not just "jump back" into my previous routines this time.

Recovering cancer patients should do a life review no matter what their age. In my case, I was 45 years old and really primed for a monumental mid-life evaluation. Everything was fair game - should I keep it, keep it as is or change it, should I pitch it, what was new that I should add? As I mentioned earlier, this process was even more difficult for me than completing chemotherapy. I don't say that to discourage you - only to give you fair notice. I wouldn't be writing about it if I didn't think the evaluation and searching process had value.

The following list includes the new additions to my life. Many of them are major lifestyle changes, such as daily meditation and exercise. These take time and a commitment to making the time to do them. Every component listed here is very meaningful and has helped me heal on multiple levels. Your list may look very different from mine, as there is more than one road to healing. I've included a lengthy list of the multiple ways different members of my support group are using to heal in the Appendix.

Don't ignore or suppress the need for full healing from your cancer experience at more than a physical level. I have chosen many of these activities because they address different levels of my healing needs. My needs were extensive because I had not really addressed them after my first two cancers. I had simply "coped". Each of you is at a different place with your recovery. Hopefully, this booklet will give you some ideas and resources to begin (or continue) your own healing journey.

- ❦ Be outside daily experiencing God's beautiful natural world. Sometimes it is only to fill the bird feeders, but I get outside daily to offer my thanks for feeling the sun, wind, or rain on my face. Good research now shows the benefits of being in nature for cancer patients.

- ❦ Breast cancer support group - monthly. I didn't join one after my first breast cancer - I don't really know why. This time, after my second breast cancer, I initially went simply for information but eventually discovered what kept me going back was the love and support, the inspiration, that I received from everyone there. Now that I'm farther along with my recovery, I am in a position to offer both "information and inspiration" to new cancer survivors.

- ❦ "Cancer Survivor's Network" - I joined the committee of a community based group of cancer survivors that planned the activities for the local 1997 National Cancer Survivors' Day event and is also working to identify and address the large unmet needs of cancer survivors in our community. We are now developing a web site, a resource guide for cancer patients, and a day-long workshop covering topics of importance to cancer survivors. This group is fun and stimulating. By developing friendships with men and women, old and young, all with different kinds of cancers, treatments, side effects, and inspirational stories to share, I have greatly broadened my horizons of understanding of both the difficulties and triumphs of being a cancer survivor.

❖ Exercise

- Walking 2-3 miles/day 5-7x/week using light wrist and ankle weights. As I mentioned previously, I was not faithful before, but now I'm outside exercising if it's above 0 degrees with no ice. Otherwise, I will use an exercise bicycle or stair stepper inside.

- T'ai Chi - daily at home. I do these slow Chinese exercises using a video as a guide. I love the slow movement, the balancing, and slowing of my thoughts during the session. I always feel centered after completing this even though I would likely obtain even more benefit if I were in a group class receiving the energy of both my classmates and my teacher.

- Chi Kung (also called Qi Gong) - daily at home and once weekly in a group with a teacher. These are also Chinese exercises however Chi Kung incorporates visualizations, and meditative breathing with the slow movements. Chi Kung was developed thousands of years before T'ai Chi with the purpose of stimulating the body's self-healing potential. I have had some very profound and unexpected metaphysical experiences doing my Chi Kung that I believe have been very instrumental with my healing. Interestingly, these happened even before I had learned that Chi Kung is used in China in their cancer clinics.

❖ Homeopathic remedies as prescribed by my homeopathic physician.

I decided to make an appointment with a homeopathic physician after doing enough reading to accept that no homeopathic remedy prescribed was likely to be harmful. I don't fully understand how homeopathy works, but I believe that it might be helpful without being harmful or outrageously expensive. I knew this physician was knowledgeable about many aspects of alternative medicine, and after talking with several people who went to him, I felt comfortable that he would be honest with me about "hope vs. hype". He also was forthright about discussing what potential dangers various alternative approaches might have for me. These homeopathic remedies listed are the ones I have taken or am currently taking. They are all very inexpensive. Although I did much of my own reading about herbs, he also has guided me in the selection of the few herbs I am taking. The calcium phosphate and silica have been prescribed to help with my osteoporosis, a side effect of early menopause, induced after my first chemotherapy at age 34.

- Cadmium sulfate 30x - for detoxification after radiation - now discontinued
- Nux vomica 30x - for detoxification after chemo - now discontinued
- Carcinosin 200x - for detoxification after chemo - 1x/week
- Calcium Phosphate 6x - for bone strengthening - 2x/day
- Silica 6x - for bone strengthening - 2x/day

❖ Meditation - daily in AM for 30-45 minutes (ideal would be 2x/day).

I do "mindful meditation" every morning before my family gets up. I learned about meditation in an 8-session class entitled "The Magic of Healing". (See resource list for information.) I have had several experiences while meditating that have positively impacted my healing. I apparently derive more benefit from meditating that I receive from the hour of sleep I give up, because I have found my body wakes up on its' own ready to meditate no matter what time I went to bed. Although I am a nutritionist to the core, *I believe that learning to meditate, and doing it faithfully, has been the most important change I have made.*

♣ Imagery

I have two sets of imagery that I do daily, which are my own visions of healing within my body. This takes 20-30 minutes daily following my meditation. I had read *Getting Well Again*, by Drs. Carl and Stephanie Simonton, when I underwent chemo in 1984. As I went through chemo the 2nd time, I found myself automatically starting to use the techniques discussed in their book for developing images of my body healing itself.

Previously I had used their "Pac-Man" image for my white blood cells seeking and destroying the cancer cells in my body. However, in 1995, I needed to change the image to something more personal to me. Swans returning in the spring have long been a symbol to me of rebirth and renewal. This time around, I preferred to image a swan, taking "Pac-Man's" place, finding cancer cells to eat and thus eliminate from my body. Later after I began meditating, I had a "vision" of flocks and flocks of swans entering my body to help with this process. In addition, now the swans were not just in my blood stream but were everywhere throughout my tissues looking for cancer cells and eliminating them. During this portion of my imagery, I visit with my swans, feed them special treats, and tell them how grateful I am for their assistance. Because there are so many swans now, I know that they will take care of me, and I don't have to worry if I miss a day of doing my visualizations.

My second set of visualizations focus on my bone marrow, the site of white blood cell production, so critical to the healthy functioning of the immune system. I visualize my bone marrow as a large beautiful English garden, filled with colorful flowers, herbs, birds, honey bees, and ponds. I am the gardener whose job it is to keep everything beautiful and healthy. I nurture the garden (my bone marrow) as I cultivate, weed, water, mulch, prune, plant, transplant, and also simply sit in the sun and enjoy its sights, smell, and sounds. It's one of my dream jobs, I love being there.

♣ Hypnotherapy

I listen to a self-guided cassette tape, individualized for me, once or twice each week before I go to sleep at night. When I wake up the next morning, I am always astounded by the sense of energy that I feel. I met a local certified hypnotherapist who works extensively with cancer patients only after the *Detroit Free Press* article was published. I am now curious whether this therapy would have helped me have more energy during chemotherapy!

♣ Feng Shui consultation and evaluation of my home.

Feng Shui is the ancient Chinese practice of assessing and altering various aspects of your physical surroundings (furniture placement, colors, aromas, shapes, etc.) in order to balance and maximize your internal energy or "Chi". This was a fun thing to do, and we are slowly making some changes in our home as a result of this consult. Some of the suggestions didn't sit well with me, but that's OK. It's important to listen to those inner feelings, too.

♣ Shiatsu

Based on traditional Chinese medicine, shiatsu is an ancient form of hands-on therapy that enlists pressure point massage and stretching to balance the flow of "Chi" throughout the body. I am intuitively drawn to many facets of Chinese healing and have just started going to a shiatsu practitioner. I have experienced relief from some physical pains but even more interesting to me have been the flashes of new insight that have occurred while having this therapy done.

♣ Prayer

I prayed before this latest cancer and chemo but, just like with my exercising, I was not faithful about it. I now pray daily, in fact many times throughout the day. I pray everyday with thankfulness for my life along with prayers for guidance and strength that I might continue to do God's plan for me. It is also very meaningful to me to be able to pray for anyone who needs prayers, which includes my clients and even total strangers. I can tell you there are no words to express what it feels like to know that people all over the country are praying for you.

♣ Reading

As strange as it may sound, I never read extensively about cancer or even the subject of cancer and nutrition during the 10+ years between my 2 breast cancers. I was immersed in a different sub-specialty field of clinical nutrition that required substantial daily reading to remain current. However, in retrospect, I suspect I was in a state of denial about my cancer history.

I've now turned my voracious appetite for knowledge to strictly reading information regarding cancer, the nutrition and cancer connections, and the books that discuss the mind-body-spirit connection. I'm now also starting to mix in more inspirational books written by cancer survivors. I certainly haven't found or had time to read all the best helpful books available. If you have a particular book to recommend, please let me know!

I have shared with you all the various new ingredients I added to my life in order to create my healing recipe. I kept many things in my life the same - my husband, Dick, and sons, Eric now 21 and Garrison now 16, my friends, pets, fun, and vacations, which have also made major contributions to my overall successful recipe for healing. My recipe is only a guide. I have found there seem to be a few ingredients that are "essential" for me while others have some leeway. My days are never identical. Yet most everything gets done to some degree.

I am now 4 full years "out" from my latest cancer diagnosis. I feel wonderful everyday, better than I ever did in the 10+ years between my two breast cancers. I have tons of energy - I never nap - I am up at 5:30 on almost all school days during the week and on the go until 11:00 each night. So far, there are no indications of a recurrence or another new cancer. Perhaps something even more astonishing is the fact that *all of my white blood cell counts have actually been within the normal range during the past 2-1/2 years* - something that was never accomplished during the 10+ years between my two breast cancers.

I have combined strategies from both medical worlds - conventional and complementary - to develop a truly integrated healing approach addressing all aspects of the mind-body-spirit connection. All the ingredients to my healing recipe have apparently worked together to create truly remarkable results. My oncologist is amazed and also impressed with the results I have been able to achieve. He even traveled to China this past year to learn more about the traditional Chinese therapies, including herbs and Chi Kung, used in China's cancer clinics in conjunction with the best of the conventional Western treatments. His hope is to learn how to combine the best of these therapies so that all cancer patients might benefit from this integrated approach to healing in the future.

This book, like my life, is a "work in progress" as I continue to fine-tune my own cancer recovery plan. There are undoubtedly many other helpful resources and therapies that also could have been included on this list. If you have read a book or tried a strategy that I have not mentioned which has been particularly helpful to you for your cancer recovery, please let me know. In addition, future and on-going research in nutrition, oncology, and alternative and complementary therapies will give us new information to incorporate into future cancer prevention, treatment, and recovery strategies.

I now understand there is no one absolute map for healing from cancer. Because each person is unique, every healing journey will be unique. I believe the seeking, the journey process itself, is as important to the ultimate healing of the person as are the various "ingredients of your own healing recipe". My hope is that this book will help you accept the challenge of being in charge of your cancer recovery and to either start your journey or help you continue on your present journey with more conviction and confidence.

The real turning point for my healing came after my first "metastatic scare" in March, 1996, approximately 6 months after finishing chemotherapy. It turned out to be "nothing", but I fell apart during the medical work-up. At that time, I finally could clearly see that my usually submerged fears of what horrible thing was coming next in my life were preventing me from both simply enjoying today and also from reaching my fullest potential as a human being. I made the decision that I could fully accept the possibility that my body might die from cancer (we still all die from something), but I was no longer going to allow cancer to kill my spirit, too - in other words, *I would not allow cancer to kill me twice!* In an instant, all my anger over this latest cancer was gone, and my fears of what's coming next in life were gone, too.

In addition, I had spent a lifetime telling myself I was extraordinarily fortunate to have survived my childhood cancer, always moving forward in life by putting a positive spin on everything and both accepting and meeting challenges with determined optimism. Finally, at this point in my recovery, I allowed myself to both identify and grieve for all the losses I also had experienced by having cancer three times. I finally cried, and cried, and cried. When I was done crying, I realized that I had done a lot of forgiving and was ready for a new life. I was well on my way to being healed.

I am incredibly blessed to still have the gift of life, and also be considered cancer free, after experiencing three separate cancer diagnoses. I now know that everything I accomplished in my life before this most recent cancer was "in spite of" my cancer history, and everything I accomplish from this point forward will be "because of" my cancer history. God must have had a plan for my life that included sharing my dietitian's knowledge and cancer experiences with other people, although it took me 47 years (almost a half a century!) to arrive at this point.

I can't foresee the future. Cancer is sneaky; it may still come back. That's OK with me. I sleep well at night knowing I'm no longer trying to outrun cancer. I'm simply trying to live each day well with a sense of contentment. The reality is, cancer or no cancer, we all have only today, in fact only this moment, to be living our life to its fullest. If cancer does return, I will be disappointed but not defeated. I believe all the changes I have made in my lifestyle have helped extend my life, although I acknowledge that fact cannot be proven. However, all the changes I have made have indisputably increased the quality of my life, a worthy goal in its own right. Finally, I know I have healed from the trauma of my cancer diagnoses, perhaps the most important benefit of all.

By sharing myself with you, I hope I've given you both "information and inspiration" to make your cancer journey meaningful. I wish you all the best for a full recovery, optimal health, and most importantly, the healing of your spirit.

⌘ APPENDIX ⌘

Therapeutic touch
Massage
Healing music during surgery
Guided imagery
Art therapy
Poetry writing
Cancer retreats
Support groups
Prayer
Relaxation
Susan Wolf Sternberg's support groups and book *A Year of Miracles*
Al Anon
Journaling
Taking one-step at a time
Exercise
Co-enzyme Q10, Pycnogenol, Aloe vera with Vitamin E
Positive thinking
Believe in your choices
Humor
Talking
Music
Yoga
Family
Friends
Essiac tea
Hydrazine sulfate
Macrobiotic diet
Ayruvedic medicine
Listening to yourself
Ritual of birthday celebrations
Reframing attitudes - victorious in cancer, not merely a survivor
Reading for information and inspiration
Any craft/art with tactile sense
Organizing family photos
Homeopathy
Meditation
Tai Chi
Chi Kung
Feng Shui
Echinacea
Astragalus
Guided imagery of cancer destruction, healing, and wellness and wholeness
Fun!
Diet changes
Birdwatching
Gardening
Belief that healing occurs at many levels and does not need to equate to a "cure".

This list shows a sample of the wide range of therapies that have been used to complement conventional treatments for cancer in order to help the whole person recover fully, to continue the journey of life in a meaningful and productive manner. Inclusion of a therapy on this list is not intended as an endorsement by the author.

❤ NUTRITION AND CANCER FATIGUE SUGGESTIONS ❤

- Give yourself permission to rest with breaks and naps whenever you need to.

- Exercise with some moderate or gentle movements everyday.
(Examples: walking, swimming, yoga, Tai Chi, Qi Gong are some suggestions)

- All treatment and disease side effects can contribute to fatigue. Tell your doctors about these symptoms so they can be treated aggressively with medical management if needed and/or complementary strategies.
(Examples: nausea, vomiting, diarrhea, pain, shortness of breath, anxiety, depression, sleep difficulty, fevers, anorexia)

- Your doctor can also evaluate if there are any additional medical reasons why you might be fatigued.

- Eat a well balanced diet with enough calories and protein.

- Make every bite count - choose nutrient dense foods and beverages.

- Use a stool in the kitchen while preparing meals (I used one in the shower, too).

- Simplify, prioritize, and delegate everything you can (my friends lovingly prepared supper for my family for 6 straight months). Give your friends recipes to prepare.

- Keep foods handy which are quick and easy to prepare. Small snacks between meals can help you achieve an adequate intake of protein and calories.

- If the fatigue is overwhelming, keep high calorie and high protein snacks in a small cooler by your sofa or bed. (This suggestion has a downside to it though because it is imperative to get up and move around frequently during the day to prevent other complications, too.)

- On days that you are feeling good, cook large batches of food and put the extra portions in the freezer.

- Eat your largest meal whenever you have the most energy during the day.

- Check to see if you qualify for Meals-on-Wheels service.

- If your food intake is inadequate, a multi-vitamin and mineral tablet may be appropriate. Check with the dietitian at your cancer center and your doctor.

- If you are having trouble consuming adequate calories and/or protein, a liquid supplement might help. Commercial products are available. Or make your own healthy shake using a recipe like "Diana's Super Soy and Phytochemical Shake".

The choices available in the health food or grocery store are overwhelming. Here are some general guidelines to help you choose a quality product.

Vitamins and Minerals:

1. Choose a supplement with the "USP" notation on the label. Having this on the label means the company is legally responsible to the FDA for meeting dissolution standards, which means the product has been tested to ensure it will actually disintegrate in your body. Additionally, this product has been tested to determine that the amounts indicated on the label are actually in the supplement and have met purity standards. Only the term "USP" guarantees that these important standards have been met.

2. The "USP" dissolution standard has not been tested with "sustained or timed release" products.

3. Check the expiration date. I have seen stores selling vitamins in a big "2 for 1" sale which were very close to the expiration date.

4. Take your vitamin or mineral supplement with food. That is especially important with fat-soluble vitamins that need to be in the presence of fat to be absorbed. (Source: Tufts University Health and Nutrition Letter, November, 1997)

Herbs and other Dietary Supplements:

Currently, there are no regulations in effect that assure consumers of either the quantity or quality of herbs or other dietary supplements being purchased. Consumer's Report has published their investigative research showing widely varying contents (quantity and purity) of various dietary supplements bought from retail stores. "Standardization" of a product is optional at this time, and indeed, there are widely differing (and contentious) views among herbalists about the pros and cons of standardizing herbs for only one active constituent. In addition, apparently even "standardized" herbs are not always what they say they are. I found two references that listed brand names of products which are reputed to "truly" supply standardized products, but I can't verify the accuracy of their reporting:

- Herbal Choice, Botalia Gold, Murdock Madaus Schwabe, Nature's Way, Eclectic Institute, Pytopharmica, Nature's Herbs, KAL
  (Source: *American Health*, Jan/Feb. 1997, page 33)

- Eclectic Institute, Nature's Herb Company, Nature's Way, Penn Herb Company, Ltd.
  (Source: *New Herbal Remedies*, by Rodale Press, 1997, page 47)

I recently learned of a trade organization called the "National Nutritional Foods Association" which requires its members who manufacture herbal and other dietary supplements to agree to random independent testing of their products for both quality and quantity as part of their "TrueLabel Program". Upon calling them, I found out they would not give me the names of their members over the telephone but suggested that I call each company to ask if they belonged to the NNFA.

This will take some legwork on your part, but may be helpful in determining if a company has enough internal quality control to be confident that outside, independent testing will verify the information they have put on the label. This industry is still evolving and hopefully will move toward defining, implementing, and enforcing standards so that consumers don't have to be in the position of "Buyer, beware", as is the unfortunate current situation. When I have called a couple of herb companies, all were willing to tell me if they belonged to the NNFA or not. All wanted to know why I was asking. If you call the companies yourself, simply say that as a consumer, you would like some indicator of quality control of the products you are choosing to buy. Conveying this information to the manufacturers will hopefully give them the message that higher and more consistent standards for the herbal industry are needed.

Some additional advice I give my clients is the importance of keeping a diary or log of all the supplements they are consuming, including brand name, dosage, frequency, along with recording any signs, symptoms, or changes they might notice that should be brought to the attention of their cancer team members. In addition, if you are starting a new complementary therapy such as acupuncture, meditation, yoga, guided imagery, etc., keep records of when you started that, too, along with any changes you observe. All of this information should be incorporated into your medical records because all of these strategies are contributing to your healing.

It is also advisable to introduce or change only one new herb, supplement, or therapy at a time. I recommend waiting 3-4 days at a minimum. That way the development of any adverse effects can be more easily traced to a particular change or addition, just like with a medication. Currently there is VERY LITTLE information available to guide practitioners regarding potential unsafe combinations of medications and herbs. If you do develop any unusual side effects or symptoms, stop your supplements and notify your physician(s) and any additional health care practitioner who is guiding you on choices of complementary therapies.

❧ CULINARY HERBS WITH ANTI-CANCER ACTIVITY ❧

Don't forget culinary herbs that may also help with the cancer prevention and cancer fighting process. Many herbs commonly used in cooking are receiving increased attention and research as their components and actions in the body are more fully understood. These herbs contain various substances ("phytochemicals") that exert their anti-cancer actions by blocking various hormone actions and metabolic pathways that are associated with the development of cancer, or they induce enzymes that help metabolize and eliminate carcinogens.

The following herbs have the highest level of anti-cancer actions:
    garlic, ginger, licorice root,
    umbelliferous (carrot) family: anise, caraway, celery, chervil, cilantro
    coriander, cumin, dill, fennel, parsley

The herbs listed next have modest level of anti-cancer actions:
    onions, flax, turmeric, mints, rosemary,
    thyme, oregano, sage, basil, tarragon

Recommendations: Increase the use of all these herbs daily in your cooking for both flavor enhancement and their phytochemical content to maximize potential cancer protective benefits. Some new interesting information concerning garlic has shown that cutting or smashing whole garlic bulbs 10 minutes before heating them helps to preserve its anti-cancer properties.

The following food items are those that I try to keep on hand at all times. Where specific brand names are mentioned, it is because I have found myself buying those products consistently for their taste and nutritional qualities. Your section of the country will likely have other or additional brands that are very good. Brands also sometimes change their contents, so I have learned to always check labels. I do most of my shopping at regular grocery stores, going to natural food or health food stores 1-2 times each month. My family eats most of this food (not all) and I do buy other healthy foods (and treats, too) for them.

❧ Produce Section:

Tofu, soft and firm
Shitake Mushrooms
Red, Yellow, and Orange Sweet Peppers
Romaine Lettuce
Carrots - baby and regular
Kale
Garlic
Onions
Apples
Red Grapefruit
Melons - any kind
Fresh Ginger
Dried apricots
Craisins

Broccoli Sprouts – *wash very thoroughly*
Broccoli and Cauliflower
Sweet potatoes
Spinach
Green onions
Winter Squash
Cabbage
Oranges
Red Grapes
Berries - any kind
Prunes
Raisins
Dried cherries

❧ My Grocery Store's "Health Food Section"

Vruit™ (100% fruit/veggie juice) - 3 pack – on the shelf
Boca Burgers® - veggie burgers in the freezer section
Soy cheese - mozzarella and cheddar – in the refrigerator section
Tempeh (White Wave) – in the refrigerator section
Baked soy squares - various flavors (White Wave) – in the refrigerator section
Silken tofu, vacuum-packed (Mori-Nu) – on the shelf
Edensoy Extra® - soy milk - Original flavor - liters and 3 pack
Dried bean soups (Health Valley) – on the shelf
Eden® pasta - look for 50-50 white/whole wheat
Eden® canned beans - look for black soybeans
Tofu dogs – in the refrigerator section
Tabouli – in the deli section
Hummus – in the deli section
Whole wheat cous-cous (Fantastic Foods) – on the shelf
Bulgur – (Bob's Red Mill ™) - on the shelf
Millet – (Bob's Red Mill™) - on the shelf

❧ Seafood/Meats

Salmon filets or steaks
Tuna filets or steaks

❧ Canned Goods

Artichoke hearts, in water
Extra Virgin olive oil
Applesauce, unsweetened
Bean soups
Salmon

Black olives
Canola Oil
Prunes, pureed - baby food
Beans, all varieties
Tuna – in water

🍎 Dry Goods and other Miscellaneous Items

Brownberry ® - Whole Wheat and Health Nut bagels
Whole wheat pita bread
Whole wheat flat bread
Whole wheat bread
All-Bran® cereal
Rolled oats - original, or quick (not instant)
Dried beans
Triscuits® - low-fat

Kashi® - The Breakfast Pilaf
Green tea
Salsa
Low-fat spaghetti sauce
Brown rice, instant
Wasa® Fiber Rye crackers

🍎 Frozen Foods

Frozen Fruit, unsweetened
Egg Substitutes
Morningstar Farms®
    Chik Nuggets™
    Breakfast Strips - bacon style
    Spicy Black Bean Burgers
Green Giant® Harvest Burgers® for Recipes™
Green Giant® Breakfast Links - Sausage Style
Freshlike® Baby Broccoli Blend – featuring Sweet Beans® (green soybeans)

Orange juice - w/calcium
Frozen veggies

🍎 Dairy Section

Organic 1% Milk
Red/Pink Grapefruit Juice

🍎 Specialty Food Store

Olive-It® - butter and olive oil spread
Better than Bouillon™ soup base

🍎 Large Chain Natural Foods Store

I buy the following items in bulk:
    Wheat bran
    Whole flax seeds
    Soy nuts

    Wheat germ
    Spices
    Tahini

Whole wheat pizza crusts
Organic milk - both liquid and dry powder
Organic yogurt - lowfat by Stonyfield Farms™
Organic butter
Organic cream cheese
Organic feta cheese
Organic eggs
Miso
Tempeh - various flavors
Baked tofu squares - various flavors
Roasted SoyButter™ (like peanut butter) by Natural Touch®
Soy flour

Feel free to photocopy this list for your own personal use. Tape it onto your refrigerator to mark those items you use up then take it with you to the grocery store.

People often ask me which fruits and vegetables are "the best" for preventing or fighting cancer. It is difficult to answer that question briefly because there are so many factors to consider. There is some research that has determined in the laboratory (test tube) which fruits and vegetables have the highest anti-oxidant activity, coming from the combined anti-oxidant activity of vitamins, minerals, and numerous phytochemicals. The following produce have the highest antioxidant activity in order of potency: (source J. Agri. Food Chem. 44:701, 3426, 1996)

- ❦ vegetables: kale, beets, red peppers, broccoli, spinach, potato, sweet potato, and corn
- ❦ fruits: blueberries and strawberries

The following have progressively lower levels:

- ❦ vegetables: cauliflower, eggplant, carrots, string beans, cabbage, squash, garlic, iceberg lettuce, celery, onion, leaf lettuce, and cucumber
- ❦ fruits: plums, oranges, red grapes, kiwi, pink grapefruit, white grapefruit, white grapes, apples, tomatoes, bananas, pears, and melons

Additional research will need to be done to validate factors regarding actual absorption of all of the phytochemicals and their impact on various metabolic activities in vivo (in real life situations, animal and human). Stay tuned in to this very exciting area.

All produce should be washed very thoroughly, even types for which the outside rind/peel is not eaten, as a knife slicing through the item could drag bacteria or other microbial contaminants onto the part you consume potentially a causing food-borne illness. This is especially important if you are still immune-suppressed. In addition, washing by scrubbing with a vegetable brush when possible or soaking in water containing a teaspoon of dish detergent/gallon of water will help reduce pesticide content on produce that cannot be scrubbed. I would not recommend eating any type of sprouts if you are still immune-suppressed.

The question of pesticides always comes up. I do agree with those who believe we derive more health benefits from eating fruits and vegetables with pesticides than from not eating fruits and vegetables. There are more than 200 studies in the scientific literature that clearly show decreased risk for many chronic diseases, including cancer, with an increased consumption of fruits and vegetables. However, I consider the issue of pesticides and their potential harmful health effects a "loose end".

So, I have chosen to selectively eat organic fruits and vegetables, using published data analyses in which fruits and vegetables were analyzed and then ranked for their content of the most potentially risky pesticides. The Environmental Working Group, a consumer-based group based in Washington, DC, has analyzed FDA pesticide inspection data from 1992 and 1993 to rate 42 fruits and vegetables and published this information on its internet site (http://www.ewg.org). They have published the information in an especially useful format. It lists the 12 most contaminated fruits and vegetables (strawberries, bell peppers and spinach tied, U.S. cherries, peaches, Mexican cantaloupe, celery, apples, apricots, green beans, Chilean grapes, cucumbers) along side alternative choices of produce which contain fewer pesticides but are also very good sources of equivalent nutrients, including phytochemicals. For one example, strawberries have a high concentration of pesticides so you may want to consider either buying organic strawberries or substituting non-organic raspberries or blueberries which contain similar nutrients and/or phytochemicals with much less contamination.

In addition, the same data have been presented in Nutrition Action Newsletter, June, 1997, ranking the pesticide content of fruits and vegetables according to a typical serving size which is also a useful tool for making decisions regarding which produce to consider buying that is organically grown. Look for this newsletter in your public library. I do not let this controversy "drive me crazy" but use the information to make informed choices about which produce to buy and eat.

❡ DINING OUT: HOW TO MAINTAIN AN ANTI-CANCER DIET ❡

Wherever I speak, the most frequently asked question I receive is, "How do you eat out and still maintain your healthful diet?" That is an excellent question and represents a common problem. Surveys have demonstrated that almost 50% of our food dollars are spent in restaurants (or for "take out" food). In addition, we are eating out an average of 3-4 times each week.

Perhaps the hardest part of modifying your diet to reduce your cancer risk is deciding what to eat while away from home. How closely you maintain your diet while eating out is up to you, and it may depend on how often you eat out (or "take out"). If you eat several meals away from home each week, or if you travel often, it may be especially important to choose wisely. Two important goals to keep in mind are minimizing your fat intake (for information on which types of fats are most harmful or beneficial, see pages 6-7 of the book) and emphasizing foods from plant sources (fruits, vegetables, grains and legumes) in your meals.

General Guidelines for Low-fat, Plant-based Eating

Choose:	Limit:
Vegetables	Meats, poultry
Garden salad	Full-fat dairy products
Mixed greens	Cream sauce
Fruit	Cheese sauce
Whole grains, starches	Hollandaise
Beans, lentils	Alfredo
Nuts, seeds	Béarnaise
Seafood (fresh or water pack)	Au gratin
Low-fat dairy	Parmigiana
Egg whites/substitutes	Croquettes
Herbs and spices	Fritters
Marinara	Filo
Tomato sauce or base	Crispy, flaky
Light wine sauce	Batter-dipped, breaded
Steamed	Deep-fried
Baked, broiled	Tempura
Grilled	Escalloped
Poached	Newburg
Roasted	Scampi
Stewed	Blackened, charbroiled
Sautéed	Smoked
Stir-fried	Lard
Olive or canola oil (< 1 tsp.)	Vegetable oil
Condiments	Condiments
Salsa	Butter, margarine
Low-fat mayo or salad dressing	Full-fat mayo or salad dressing
Vinegar	Full-fat sour cream
Lemon juice	Full-fat cream cheese
Soy sauce	"Special sauce"
Cocktail sauce	Tartar sauce
Ketchup	Guacamole
Barbecue/steak sauce	
Mustard	
Pickle relish	
Pepper	
Jam/syrup/honey	

Helpful Tips

- Think "Ethnic": Ethnic restaurants are more likely to offer a wide variety of plant-based menu items. Chinese, Mexican, and Italian are the most common ethnic choices in the U.S., but many larger cities also offer Indian, Middle Eastern, Japanese, Thai, Korean, or Ethiopian fare. Challenge yourself to try new foods!

- Have a Plan: To select a restaurant, look in the Yellow Pages of the phone book or ask friends or family members (or, if you are traveling, a hotel manager or desk clerk) for suggestions. If you are trying a new restaurant, call ahead to ask what low fat or vegetarian choices they offer or would be willing to prepare. You can also pick up a copy of their menu, ask them to fax it to you, or simply read over the menu before being seated. Frequent travelers may want to order a copy of Vegetarian Journal's Guide to Natural Foods Restaurants in the US and Canada (see references).

- Make the Best of it: If you are traveling and have limited restaurant choices (for example, at a rest stop on the highway), try to find a chain or fast food restaurant that you know offers menu items which fit into your healthy diet. The Vegetarian Resource Group has some very helpful guides for anyone who is trying to eat vegetarian at fast food or chain restaurants (see references).

- Be Creative: Even if there are no entrées on the menu that fit into your diet, you may be able to create a healthy meal out of several side dishes, appetizers, or soup and salad. Many salad bars offer a variety of healthy items. You may want to see what is available at the salad bar before you order.

- Share/Save the Sinful: If you can't resist ordering an entrée or a dessert that does not fit into your healthy diet, see if someone will share it with you. Then order a healthy entrée and/or salad or soup to go with it. If you will be dining alone, ask for a doggie bag (or box) and save the rest for later.

- Bring Your Own: If you're going someplace where you're not sure what you'll find to eat, or if you're headed to a junk food haven, bring your own healthy meals or snacks in your briefcase, purse, or backpack (see "Travel Tips" for suggestions for what to bring). Store food in a cooler for longer outings or vacations. If you'll be staying in a hotel, call ahead to ask if there will be a mini fridge in your room. This will give you more options for keeping your own food on hand.

- Just Ask: If you are unsure whether or not an item is vegetarian or if you would like to know how something is prepared, ask your server. He or she should either be able to tell you or find out for you. It may be harder to get information from fast food restaurants, although some, such as Subway and Wendy's, do provide nutritional information right in the store. If you still have questions, you can ask the manager for the phone number of the chain's corporate headquarters.

- Make a Request: Most any restaurant will respond to requests to modify an item, for example leaving the butter off your vegetables, putting your salad dressing on the side, or leaving the meat or dairy out of certain dishes. You may want to emphasize that these requests are for your health. At some of the more upscale restaurants, the chef may be able to prepare a special meal for you, such as a vegetable stir-fry or a tomato-based pasta dish with vegetables. If possible, you may want to call the restaurant ahead of time to make a special request, especially during busy times (i.e. Friday or Saturday night). If the restaurants you frequent have a limited selection of healthy items, encourage them to offer more choices.

Hidden Fat Traps and Vegetarian Concerns

- Refried beans often contain lard. Be sure to ask.
- Many soups, such as vegetable and bean soups, and rice dishes which appear to be vegetarian contain meat, meat stock, or animal fat.
- Some house salads are served with bacon bits, cheese, or egg. You should be able to order your salad without one or all of these items.
- Many sauces, including pasta and even pizza sauces, may contain meat, cheese, meat stocks, or animal fats. *When in doubt, ask!*

Salad Bar Tips

- Emphasize dark greens (romaine, spinach) vs. iceberg
- Load up on fruit (fresh if available)
- Top salads with a variety of veggies (shredded carrots, bell peppers, tomatoes, broccoli, cauliflower, cucumbers, mushrooms, green peas, sprouts, etc.)
- Add some garbanzo beans, kidney beans, and/or sunflower seeds for extra fiber and protein
- Skip the creamy, full-fat dressings and choose low-fat or fat-free dressing or a small amount of oil--preferably olive or canola--and vinegar. Or try substituting lemon juice or salsa with some pepper.
  Suggestion: Carry a very small container of olive oil in your purse, briefcase, or backpack to use with vinegar on your salad.
- Avoid or limit creamy mixed salads such as potato salad, pasta salads, and coleslaw

Beverage Suggestions

- Water or mineral water with a slice of fruit
- Fruit/vegetable juices
- Iced tea
- Hot tea (green, herbal, black)
- Milk (low-fat or skim)
- Soy milk (from home)

Suggestion: If you drink coffee, add skim or low-fat milk instead of cream, or drink it black.

Meal Suggestions for a Low-Fat, Plant-Based Diet

- Asian - Examples are Chinese, Korean, Japanese, Thai, Vietnamese and Mongolian, which vary significantly. There should be many choices that emphasize vegetables and/or tofu. *Request minimal oil or steamed for all dishes.*

Miso soup	Sushi (can be ordered vegetarian),
Steamed vegetable spring rolls	Steamed rice (brown if available) or pasta
Mu Shu with vegetables or seafood	Spicy tofu, vegetables, or seafood
Steamed vegetable dumplings (pot stickers)	California rolls
Cabbage or mixed green salads (with minimal or no oil)	
Teriyaki fish with vegetables	
Broth-based soups with vegetables, seaweed, seafood, rice or noodles	
Brown, Szechuan, Hunan, black bean or garlic sauce	
Stir-fried or steamed vegetables and bean curd (tofu) or seafood	
Fresh fruit	Green or oolong tea

Avoid/Limit: Fried egg rolls, wontons, fried rice and noodles, dishes which emphasize meat--especially duck, beef, or pork, egg foo young, deep fried or breaded and fried dishes, tempura, dishes with coconut milk, teas made with cream or whole milk.

- <u>Italian</u>

Bread with a touch of olive oil
Raw vegetables
Bean salads
Green salad with olive oil and vinegar or low-fat dressing on the side
Lentil or minestrone soup (may contain meat/meat stock)
Pasta e fagioli (pasta and beans, note: may not be vegetarian)
Pasta with marinara, tomato, or wine sauce or small amounts of pesto sauce
Pasta primavera (with tomato or wine--not cream--base)
Steamed or baked (not fried) eggplant or zucchini with tomato sauce

Fresh fruit
Steamed or roasted vegetables
Seafood cacciatore

Avoid/Limit: Buttered garlic bread, meatballs, Italian sausage, veal dishes, pasta stuffed with meats or cheeses, cream sauces such as Alfredo or carbonara, sauces with meat or cheese, parmigiana or breaded and fried meats or vegetables.

- <u>Mexican</u>

Green salad
Fresh fruit
Veggie or seafood fajita
Spanish rice
Gazpacho - request no sour cream or have it on the side
Bean, vegetable, or seafood enchilada (with tomato-based—not cheese—sauce)
Refried beans (make sure they're not cooked in lard or fat)
Huevos rancheros (small portion—i.e. one egg—without cheese)
Peppers--all varieties
Toppings: salsa, salsa verde, picante sauce, lettuce, tomato, peppers, onions, small amounts of guacamole

Steamed vegetables
Bean burrito
Bean taco or tostada
Black beans (may come as a side dish)

Avoid/Limit: Fried tortilla chips, taco salads, beef tacos, deep-fried tacos or tortillas (chimichangas), chili con carne, sausage, fried chile rellenos, full-fat cheeses and cheese sauces, full-fat sour cream, deep fried ice cream.

- <u>Indian</u> - Nepalese food is similar. There should be many choices which emphasize vegetables, legumes, and herbs

Vegetable raita salads (usually made with cucumbers and yogurt)
Mixed vegetable salads
Dahl (lentil) dishes
Basmati rice with vegetables
Vegetable biryani
Aloo ghobi
Masala sauce
Fresh fruit

Chapati and naan bread (not fried)
Tomato-based dishes
Saffron rice
Vegetable curries
Steamed vegetable dumplings
Chutneys (mango, onion, or mint)
Chai made with skim or soy milk

Avoid/Limit: Samosas, pakoras, dishes which emphasize meat--especially beef or lamb, heavy cream sauces, dishes cooked with butter or ghee, paneer (Indian cheese), fried breads, lassi (sweet yogurt drink), chai made with cream or whole milk.

- <u>Middle Eastern</u> - Should offer plenty of vegetable- and lentil-based entrees

Greek salad (without feta, or ask for a small amount of feta on the side)
Grape leaves (stuffed with rice, tomato and onion. Note: some may have meat)

Lentil or black bean soup	Fattoush salad
Tomato and cucumber salads	Tabouli
Rice	Pita bread (whole wheat if available)
Baba ghanouj	Hummus
Mujadara	Baked (not fried) falafel
Vegetable moussaka	Vegetable boreks
Dried fruit	

Avoid/Limit: Meat dishes, high-fat (filo) spinach pies, deep-fried falafel, baklava.

- <u>American, European, or Bar and Grill</u>

Garden or side salad--ask for low-fat dressing on the side or oil and vinegar
Steamed vegetables (some are prepared with butter or creamy sauces)
Soups: Broth/tomato based, vegetable, lentil or bean (may not be vegetarian)
Veggie sandwich or roll-up (some have cheese or mayo)
Egg white or egg substitute omelet--no cheese, lots of veggies
Pizza with no cheese or "half the cheese" and veggies (see "Pizza Place" suggestions)
Baked potato--try salsa as a topping instead of sour cream and butter

Pasta with marinara sauce	Stir-fried vegetables with rice or pasta
Grilled, broiled or poached salmon or tuna	Veggie burger
Rice pilaf (may not be vegetarian)	Raw vegetables
Fruit	Low- or non-fat yogurt or sorbet

Avoid/Limit: Large portions of meat, especially red meats--such as hamburgers, sausages or ham, full-fat cheeses and cheese sauces, cream sauces, most fried foods (especially deep-fried or breaded and fried), and high-fat condiments (see "General Guidelines").

- <u>Pizza Places/Sub Shops</u>

Garden or side salad (order without cheese or meat)
Greek salad (without feta cheese or dressing, or a small amounts on the side)
Pizza: Get hand-tossed or thin crust, not deep-dish or pan-fried
    Get a cheeseless pizza, or ask for "light" cheese or "half the cheese"
    Add lots of veggies, such as broccoli, green peppers, tomatoes, spinach, onions, olives, mushrooms, and artichoke hearts. Also try pineapple!
Pasta with marinara sauce (may not be vegetarian)
Vegetarian sub with no cheese or "half the cheese," light mayo or dressing (or mustard) and lots of veggies
Veggie "pizza" sub with no cheese or "half the cheese" and lots of veggies
Tuna sub made with low-fat mayo or dressing, and lots of veggies
Suggestion: If you want meat on your sub, stick with a lower-fat choice such as turkey or chicken breast, and ask for half the standard amount of meat (and cheese) and extra veggies.

Avoid/Limit: Buttery/cheesy bread sticks, buttered garlic bread, French fries (especially chili cheese fries), chef salads, potato/snack chips, meat toppings on pizza, meat subs—especially "Italian," ham, salami, meatball, and steak subs, ribs, chicken wings, pasta dishes with meats/cheeses, most desserts.

- Delis/Bagel Shops

Garden or side salad
Vegetarian Grape leaves
Bean or lentil salads
Tabouli
Greek salad (without feta cheese, or a small amount of feta on the side)
Low-fat or fat-free salad dressing or small amount of oil with vinegar
Pasta, potato, rice, or tofu salads made with low-fat dressings
Cooked seasoned vegetables (not in creamy or oily sauces)
Soups: Broth- or tomato-based vegetable, lentil or bean (may not be vegetarian)
Sandwiches:
    Bread, bagel, pita or roll (wheat or whole grain if available)
    Vegetarian (with no cheese or "half the cheese")
    Hummus
    Tuna made with low-fat mayo or dressing
    Lots of veggies (lettuce, tomatoes, peppers, onions, olives, etc.)
    Low-fat mayo or dressing, mustard
Suggestion: If you want meat on your sandwich, stick with a lower-fat choice such as turkey or chicken breast, and ask for half the standard amount of meat (and cheese) and extra veggies.
Spaghetti with marinara sauce
Hot baked potatoes (plain)
Soft pretzel with mustard
Low-fat yogurt
Low-fat frozen yogurt with fresh fruit

Notes:
At grocery stores these items may be found behind the deli counter or prepackaged in cases near the deli. Some items may be located elsewhere in the store, such as near the produce section.
Be sure to check dates on prepackaged items before buying them. Also, feel free to ask the deli server for suggestions (what is fresh, what they recommend, etc.) before you order.
For other healthy grocery items, check for a "health food" section. Soy products, such as soy milk and baked tofu, and organic dairy products are now available in many "mainstream" grocery stores.
Many grocery store delis are now featuring take-out meals. Be sure to check ingredient labels, as many of these items are not low fat. For example, potatoes may be mashed with whole milk and butter, or twice baked with cheese and sour cream.

Avoid/Limit: Full-fat creamy potato or pasta salads and coleslaws, chef salads, potato/snack chips, sandwiches with meat—especially bacon, salami, pastrami, ham and cheese, or corned beef, and most desserts and baked goods, including brownies, cheesecake, cookies, croissants, and regular (full-fat) muffins.

- Breakfast/Bakeries – breakfast bars may have a variety of old cererals and fresh fruit

Oatmeal (or other whole-grain hot cereals)--with low/non-fat milk, or soy milk (bring from home)
Cold cereals--whole grain, such as Raisin Bran®, All Bran®, Wheaties®, or Cheerios®
Low-fat fruit or bran muffin
Fresh fruit and fruit juices
Dry wheat toast with or without jam—ask for no butter
Bagel or English muffin with or without jam—ask for no butter
Pancakes or waffles without butter (may contain eggs and dairy)--with fruit
Egg white or egg substitute omelets—ask for no cheese, lots of veggies
Roasted or boiled potatoes (ask if there is added fat)
Low-fat yogurt

Avoid/Limit: Bacon, ham, sausage, large omelets with meats/cheeses, quiches, croissants, regular (full-fat) muffins, deep-fried French toast, granola (unless it's low fat), whole milk, cream, hash browns, fried potatoes.

- Fast Food

Garden or side salad (without cheese) with fat free or low-fat dressing (Note: Many are mainly iceberg lettuce, which is low in nutrients and cancer-fighting phytochemicals)
Baked potato (no cheese sauce, or cheese sauce on the side) with broccoli and/or salsa
Bean burrito or taco--ask for beans instead of beef, no cheese, and extra veggies
Low-fat submarine sandwiches (see "Sub Shop" suggestions above)
Low-fat bagel sandwiches (see "Bagel Shop" suggestions above)
Veggie pita--no added sauce, or low-fat sauce on the side
Burgerless burger (bun, lettuce, onions, extra tomatoes, ketchup and mustard, with or without cheese and mayo or special sauce)
Grilled or broiled chicken sandwich with low-fat sauce or sauce on the side
Pasta bar--choose tomato-based sauces, avoid meat/cheese/cream sauces
Salad bar--See "Salad Bar Tips" (below), avoid chef salads, taco salads, and regular (full-fat) salad dressings

Fast Food Breakfast Options:
    Low-fat bran muffin
    Cereal (such as Cheerios®) with low-fat milk (or soy milk from home)
    English muffin with or without jam—ask for no butter
    Pancakes with syrup (may contain eggs and dairy)—ask for no butter
    Low-fat yogurt
    Orange or other fruit juice

Avoid/Limit: Burgers--especially double or quarter-pound burgers, deep-fried chicken or fish sandwiches, chicken nuggets, mayo, cheese, cheese sauce, special sauce, sour cream, French fries, snack chips, whole milk, milkshakes made with whole milk or oil, most (especially deep-fried) desserts, breakfast pastries, egg/meat biscuits, super size or deluxe meals.

- Gas Stations/Convenience Stores - Although some convenience stores may have prepackaged sandwiches, they usually don't have many healthy choices for meals. If you do stop at a convenience store for snacks, here are some of the better choices:

Mixed nuts, cashews, peanuts, sunflower seeds or pumpkin seeds (dry roasted if available)
Fig bars (fat free if available)
Dried fruit
Low-fat, whole grain crackers
Low-fat "breakfast" or granola bars
Pretzels
Whole grain cereals
Fruit/vegetable juices

Sample Menus

The following menus were designed to provide suggestions for maintaining a low-fat, plant-based diet for those times when your only meal choices may be chain or fast food restaurants. They represent some of the best choices available from a limited selection of healthy menu items.

Day 1: Chain Restaurants:

<u>Breakfast: Big Boy's</u>

Bowl of oatmeal--skim milk on side (or bring your own soy milk)
Fresh strawberries
Wheat toast (no butter) with jam
Grapefruit juice

<u>Lunch: Olive Garden</u>

Capellini Pomodoro (angel hair pasta with tomatoes and Romano cheese)
Minestrone soup
Plain breadstick (ask for no butter)
Ice water

<u>Dinner: Applebee's</u>

Low-Fat Veggie Quesadilla (comes with non-fat cheese and sour cream)
Steamed broccoli and carrots (special request)
Hot or iced tea

<u>Snacks: from home or grocery</u>

1 peeled orange
2 T. roasted soy nuts or soy nut butter
10 whole grain crackers
8 oz. soy drink box
Plenty of fresh water

Nutritional Value:

Provides approximately 4 servings of fruits, 5 servings of vegetables, 10 servings of grains (including 2 whole grains), and 2-3 servings of soy.

Provides approximately 2000 calories, 90 grams of protein, 40 grams of fat, 30 grams of fiber, and 18 % of calories from fat.

Note: Items may be added or deleted to meet higher or lower calorie needs.

Day 2: Fast Food Restaurants:

Breakfast: McDonald's
Lowfat Apple Bran Muffin
Cheerios® with 1% milk (or bring your own soy milk)
Large orange juice

Lunch: Wendy's
Garden Veggie Pita, no added dressing
Fruit juice

Dinner: Subway
Veggie Delite™ 12" Sub—without cheese
Iced or hot tea or water

Snacks-from home or grocery
1/2 c. carrot sticks or baby carrots
1 apple
8 oz. soy drink box
2 T. roasted soy nuts
Plenty of fresh water

Nutritional Value:
Provides approximately 4 servings of fruits, 4-5 servings of vegetables, 13 servings of grains (10 whole grains), and 2-3 servings of soy.
Provides approximately 1850 calories, 60 grams of protein, 30 grams of fat, 25 grams of fiber, and 15 % of calories from fat.

Travel Tips - Ideas for Eating on the Road or Bringing Your Own Food

Whole grain bread or bagels (for sandwiches)
Instant or prepared hummus, for sandwiches or a veggie dip (should be kept cold once prepared)
Soy nut butter, to spread on sandwiches, crackers, or fruit
Small cans of beans with pop-up lids
Small cans of water-pack tuna with pop-up lids
Fresh veggies such as baby carrots, carrot sticks or pepper slices
Fresh fruits, such as bananas, apples, pears, oranges, peaches, nectarines or plums
Small cans of fruit (preferably in fruit juice or "lite" syrup) with pop-up lids
Fresh fruit salad (store in air-tight container)
Dried fruits, such as raisins, figs, or apricots
Cups of low-fat or soy yogurt (keep cold)
Small boxes of whole grain cold cereals
Nutlettes Plus® cereal--makes its own soy milk (see references for order info.)
Instant cups of soup
Instant cups of hot whole grain cereal
Low-fat, whole-grain muffins or quickbreads—such as pumpkin or banana (homemade)
Popcorn--preferably air-popped or popped in olive or canola oil
Low-fat, whole grain crackers or pretzels
Roasted soy nuts
Dry-roasted nuts or seeds
Soy drink boxes
Fruit/vegetable juices
Plenty of fresh water
Iced tea and/or tea bags to make hot tea
Small container of olive oil for salad dressing and/or bread in restaurants that only have vegetable oil

You may want to stop at grocery stores along the way to pick up extra snacks, or healthy meals from the deli or salad bar. Farmers' markets or roadside stands are also good places to stock up on fresh fruits and veggies. Bring whatever you will need for preparation or consumption of your meals (i.e. cutting knife, utensils, napkins, plates or bowls, cups or mugs, storage containers).

Airlines: The Vegetarian Resource Group (see references) recommends requesting a special meal when you make your reservation and then again 24 hours before your flight is scheduled to leave. Choices may include bland-soft, diabetic, Kosher, low fat, low sodium, low cholesterol, vegetarian with dairy, vegan (no eggs or dairy), or fruit plate. Some international flights also offer special ethnic meals, which may include additional vegetarian options. The best choices for a low-fat, plant-based meal will most likely be vegan, fruit plate, or vegetarian ethnic options. Another option is to bring your own meal or snacks. It's a good idea to do this anyway, to ensure that you'll have something to eat in case, for whatever reason, you don't get your meal. Also, be sure to stay well hydrated; take advantage of the beverage service or bring your own water or other non-caffeinated beverages, such as fruit or vegetable juices.

Special Note: If you will be crossing international borders, be sure to check on regulations for bringing food into the country.

Conclusion

Once you begin to learn what choices are available at various restaurants, and what the healthiest options are, the task of maintaining your anti-cancer diet while eating out should become easier. You may even find that it is fun to experiment with new foods at ethnic restaurants! Although it is certainly a challenge to find healthy foods while eating out, it doesn't have to be a chore. Check out some of the resources listed on page 48 for further suggestions. Happy (and healthy) dining!

This chapter, "Dining Out: How to Maintain Your Anti-Cancer Diet", was written in 1998 by Sara Post, MPH, as part of her graduate studies at The University of Michigan under the supervision of Diana Dyer, MS, RD.

✿ RESOURCES ✿

✿ *Cancer*

Love, Susan, M., M.D., *Dr. Susan Love's Breast Book*, Addison-Wesley Publishing, 2nd edition, 1995. **The "Bible" of information needed by breast cancer patients to intelligently talk to their doctors and make informed decisions.**

Love, Susan, M., M.D., *Dr. Susan Love's Hormone Book*, Random House, New York, 1997. I include this book here because of the author's thorough discussion of the controversies regarding hormone replacement therapy after having breast cancer, herbs that have estrogenic properties, along with information about the possible benefits, the unknowns and concerns regarding the use of soy for breast cancer patients.

Morra, Marion and Eve Potts, *Choices - The New, Most up-to-date Sourcebook for Cancer Information*, Avon Books, 1994. A very good resource although 1994 now seems "old".

Murphy, G.P., M.D., L.B. Morris, and D. Lange, The American Cancer Society's book, *Informed Decisions: The Complete Book of Cancer Diagnosis, Treatment, and Recovery*, Viking Publishers, New York, 1997. An encyclopedia-type book on everything you want to know about cancer. Although the book is huge, you can pick and choose sections to read that are relevant for you.

✿ *Alternative Medicine*

Chopra, Deepak, MD - any of his books, although the one I chose to read first, *Quantum Healing*, was too difficult for me to read as a starting point. I needed to read it twice, with 6 months and several other books under my belt between readings. Then the ideas in this book made more sense to me.

Collinge, William, M.P.H., Ph.D., *The American Holistic Health Association Complete Guide to Alternative Medicine*, Warner Books, New York, 1996 - good overview, includes multiple references, and each chapter concludes with the strengths and limitations of the particular therapy being discussed and guidelines on choosing a practitioner for that therapy.

Eisenberg, DM, et al., "Unconventional Medicine in the United States - Prevalence, Costs, and Patterns of Use", New England Journal of Medicine 328 (4):246-252, 1993. The article that really gave a "wake-up call" to U.S. medical clinicians regarding the extent of use of various aspects of alternative medicine being used by their patients without informing their doctors.

Fugh-Berman, Adriane, M.D., *Alternative Medicine: What Works - A Comprehensive, Easy-to-Read Review of the Scientific Evidence, Pro and Con*, Odonian Press, Tucson, Arizona, 1996. A very good easy-to-read overview (not just of cancer) aimed at the layperson, medical professional, and researcher, includes multiple scientific references.

Kabat-Zinn, Jon, Ph.D., *Full Catastrophe Living*, Delacorte Press, New York, 1990. There are zillions of books on meditation. This is one that explains it well and gives many case examples of how the incorporation of mindful meditation into daily life has improved the health of average Americans. Helpful cassette tapes developed by the author are also available.

"The Magic of Healing - from Prevention to Renewal" - The Eight Step Guide to Physical, Mental and Spiritual Well-Being. Developed by Drs. Deepak Chopra and David Simon. This is the course I took where I learned to meditate along with other aspects of Ayruvedic medicine. Available by certified instructors around the country. Call 1-800-757-8897 for more information.

Micozzi, MS, M.D., Ph.D., *Fundamentals of Complementary and Alternative Medicine*, Churchill Livingstone, Inc., 1996 - very good in-depth explanations of the various alternative healing traditions with many scientific references for further reading.

Moyers, Bill, *Healing and the Mind*, Doubleday Publishers, 1993 - the video is also available as seen on PBS in 1993, audio tapes, and resource guide by calling 1-800-336-1917, or write P.O. Box 2284, S. Burlington, VT 05407. A wonderful, inspirational, and award-winning PBS series. If you haven't seen it, get the tapes from the library.

Murray Michael, N.D., and Joseph Pizzorno, N.D., *Encyclopedia of Natural Medicine*, Prima Publishing, Rocklin, CA, 1991. An extensively referenced book of the principles and applications of natural medicine by two naturopathic physicians from Bastyr University, a naturopathic college in Seattle, WA, that also has both an American Dietetic Association approved Dietetics undergraduate degree and a Dietetic Internship. These authors have co-written several other books, too.

"Qi - The Journal of Traditional Eastern Health and Fitness", A quarterly journal to educate the public about the benefits of Asian traditions of healing. Recommended by my Chi Kung instructor as a resource for finding qualified Tai Chi and Chi Kung instructors in your locality. Available at some large book stores or phone # 1-800-787-2600.

Weil, Andrew, MD, *Spontaneous Healing - How to Discover and Enhance Your Body's Natural Ability to Maintain and Heal Itself*, Alfred A. Knopf, 1995. An overview with case examples of alternative approaches to healing and maintaining optimal health. Easy to read. A very good book to start exploring in this field, although if you choose to adopt all the recommendations in his book, you'll agree with me that there is nothing "spontaneous" about your improved health. His plan requires a commitment to lifestyle changes, effort, and time (hence the title for his newest book, *Eight Weeks to Optimum Health,* and even 8 weeks is optimistic!).

● *Alternative Cancer Treatments*

Austin, S, N.D., and C Hitchcock, MSW, *Breast Cancer: What You Should Know (but may not be told) about Prevention, Diagnosis, and Treatment*, Prima Publishing, Rocklin, CA, 1994 - a very interesting synthesis of both medical and alternative information as a naturopathic physician (SA) tries to help his wife (CH) choose her treatments after being diagnosed with breast cancer. For the most part, it is balanced and thoughtful book.

Boik, J, *Cancer and Natural Medicine - A Textbook of Basic Science and Clinical Research*, Oregon Medical Press, 1996. THE textbook I was looking for - gives a very good introduction to the steps of the carcinogenic process and very detailed information on the research that has shown how various nutrients and "natural products" may effect this process. The author is an engineer who is also trained in acupuncture and Chinese herbal medicine. There is nothing else like this book available that I've seen. Those without an extensive medical and/or nutritional background will need to frequently use a medical dictionary.

Boik, John, and Keith Block, M.D. are jointly publishing a new book entitled *A Patient's Guide to Natural Medicines for Cancer* - expected publication in 1999. Based on the thorough approach Mr. Boik took with his other book, I am hoping for the same attention to accurate detail in a more "user-friendly" book for patients with cancer.

Cassileth, BR, and CC Chapman, "Alternative and Complementary Cancer Therapies", Cancer 77 (6):1026-1034, 1996. Good overview in the mainstream medical press.

Lerner, Michael, Ph.D., *Choices in Healing - Integrating the Best of Conventional and Complementary Approaches to Cancer*, MIT Press, 1994. **The BEST resource I've currently found that fairly and thoroughly discusses many, but not all, unproven therapies for cancer.** This entire book is on the internet at the following URL (http://www.commonwealhealth.org/canproj.html) and is currently being updated. I recommend this book to all of my clients.

♠ *Herbs*

Craig, Winston, Ph.D., RD, *The Use and Safety of Common Herbs and Herbal Teas,* Golden Harvest Books, Berrian Springs, MI, 1996. A good overview.

Duke, James, Ph.D., *The Green Pharmacy,* Rodale Press, 1997. Fun to read. This book unfortunately has no references, but Dr. Duke is a highly-respected botanist by both the academic and herbal communities.

German Government's "Commission E Monographs" on herbs and their efficacy and safety, etc., have been recently been translated into English by The American Botanical Council. This information is considered the world's largest compilation of data supporting the safe and appropriate indications for using medicinal plants (order by calling 1-800-373-7105).

"Herbalgram" - The peer-reviewed journal of the American Botanical Council and the Herb Research Foundation - two very responsible organizations promoting accurate scientific research and education of the public about medicinal benefits and potential of herbs. Can be found at large bookstores, natural food stores and even some grocery stores. Published quarterly.

Keville, Kathi, *Herbs for Health and Healing,* St. Martin's Press, 1996 - good section on cautions and considerations.

The Review of Natural Products (formerly The Lawrence Review of Natural Products) - an extensive series of unbiased, peer-reviewed, and referenced reviews of natural products that includes information on botany, history, chemistry, pharmacology, toxicology, summary, and references. Published by Facts and Comparisons, Wolters Kluwer Company, 111 West Port Plaza, Suite 300, St. Louis, MO, 63146-3098.

Taylor, Nadine, MS, RD, *Green Tea: The Natural Secret for a Healthier Life,* Kensington Books, 1998. A well-researched book.

Tyler, Varro, Ph.D., Sc.D., *Herbs of Choice - The Therapeutic Use of Phytomedicinals,* Haworth Press, 1994 - a very thorough explanation of the clinical research on medicinal effects of herbs. Dr. Tyler (now retired from Purdue University) is considered "the" leading scientific expert in this country promoting the safe and appropriate medicinal use of herbs. Organized by therapeutic indication - disease and/or organ function. (new edition now available)

Tyler, Varro, Ph.D., Sc.D.,*The Honest Herbal: a Sensible Guide to the Use of Herbs and Related Remedies,* Pharmaceutical Products Press, New York, 3rd edition, 1993. Organized by herb. (new edition now available)

Weed, Susun S., *Breast Cancer? Breast Health: The Wise Woman Way,* Ash Tree Publishing, Woodstock, NY, 1996. The author is a highly esteemed herbalist within the herbal community. The book is extensively referenced in the manner I prefer (specific vs. general). I strongly agree with her emphasis on the importance of whole foods vs. supplements. I expect to learn much about herbs and their uses from this book.

❧ Cancer Survivorship

Anderson, Greg, *50 Essential Things to do When the Doctor Says It's Cancer,* Plume Publishers, 1993. **The best book to buy a friend early after their diagnosis.** Each chapter is very short and succinct - easy to read when you're in a state of shock and/or simply frazzled.

Canfield, J, MV Hansen, P Aubery, and N Mitchell, RN, *Chicken Soup for the Surviving Soul,* Health Communications, Inc., Deerfield Beach, FL, 1996. A wonderful, hopeful, inspirational book. Buy it for a friend or relative with cancer.

Halvorsen-Boyd, Ph.D., Glenna and Lisa Hunter, Ph.D., *Dancing in Limbo - Making Sense of Life after Cancer*, Jossey-Bass Publishers, San Francisco, 1995. A very good description of the various stages of recovery, based on the personal experiences of both authors.

Harwell, Amy, *When Your Friend Gets Cancer - How You Can Help,* Harold Shaw Publishers, Wheaton, Illinois, 1987. **The best book to buy yourself when you have a friend with cancer.**

National Coalition for Cancer Survivorship, Hoffman, Barbara, Editor, *A Cancer Survivor's Almanac - Charting Your Journey*, Chronimed Publishing, 1996 - **the best guide for "seasoned survivors"** - would be overwhelming on the day of diagnosis.

Siegel, Bernie S., MD, *Love, Medicine, and Miracles* - Dr. Siegel's first book. Many cancer patients say this book was a life-saver. However, it is intense, and not every patient is ready early after their diagnosis to delve into his questions. Additionally, this book has been highly criticized by some cancer patients who believe Dr. Siegel is indirectly stating cancer patients' own negative thoughts and emotions may be "causing" their own cancers, although I didn't read it that way.

Siegel, Bernie S., M.D., *Peace, Love, and Healing - Bodymind Communication and the Path to Self-Healing: An Exploration*, Harper and Row, New York, 1989. Dr. Siegel's second book, an extension of his first.

Sternberg, Susan Wolf, *A Year of Miracles - A Healing Journey from Cancer to Wholeness,* Star Mountain Press, Ann Arbor, MI, 1996. This is an incredibly inspirational book written by a cancer survivor diagnosed with widely metastatic kidney cancer who sought out and combined the best that conventional and complementary medicine could offer her. She is alive and thriving 8+ years after her diagnosis!

❧ Cancer and Nutrition

"Eating Hints for Cancer Patients", National Institutes of Health, National Cancer Institute - currently being revised. Ask your cancer center for a free copy or call 1-800-4-CANCER.

Nixon, Daniel, MD, *The Cancer Recovery Eating Plan - The Right Foods to Help Fuel Your Recovery*, Times Books, 1996. Overall, this is an informative and hopeful book with wonderful, healthful recipes.

Weihofen, MS, RD, and C. Marino, MD, *The Cancer Survival Cookbook*, Chronimed Publishing, 1998. A wide selection of helpful recipes and information from the oncology dietitian at The University of Wisconsin Comprehensive Cancer Center.

Keane, M, MS, and D. Chase, MS, *The What to Eat if You Have Cancer Cookbook,* Contemporary Books, 1997. A very good chapter on shakes and smoothies.

"American Institute of Cancer Research Newsletter", AICR, 1759 R Street NW, Washington, D.C., 20009 - free information, recipes, and newsletter focusing on cancer and nutrition. This privately funded research and education organization has been a pioneer in the area of nutrition and cancer. All their educational information is based on "cutting edge" research, their quarterly newsletters are packed with wonderful recipes and research updates. It is all available free of charge, although of course they hope for contributions. I've given money to them for many years. **Get on their mailing list** by calling 1-800-843-8114.

World Cancer Research Fund and The American Institute for Cancer Research, *Food, Nutrition and the Prevention of Cancer: a Global Perspective*, AICR, 1997. Extensive information.

Sattilaro, A. J., M.D., *Recalled by Life,* Avon Books, New York, NY, 1982. A physician's own story of his cancer diagnosis and subsequent change to a macrobiotic diet that he is convinced substantially extended his life. (He did subsequently die of recurrent cancer.) I did not choose to go the full macrobiotic route, but this is the book that actually got me thinking seriously about making changes in my diet.

The American Dietetic Association can offer assistance in the following ways:

Dietitian Referral Phone Line - 1-800-366-1655
Dietitian Referral Internet Site - http://www.eatright.org
Dial-A-Dietitian - 1-900-CALL-AN-RD - speak directly to a Registered Dietitian - charges of $1.95 for the first minute and then $0.95 for each subsequent minute begin after you begin discussion with the dietitian.

♣ *Newsletters to which I Subscribe*

National Alliance of Breast Cancer Organizations, 9 East 37th Street, 10th Floor, New York, New York 10016
National Breast Cancer Coalition, 1707 L Street, NW, Suite 1060, Washington, DC 20036
"The Network News" - National Women's Health Network, 514 10th Street, N.W., Suite   400, Washington, D.C. 20004
"Women's Health Advocate" Newsletter, 10310 Main Street #301, Fairfax VA 22030
"Cancer Outlook" (published by Scientific American Publications), Dept. C., P.O. Box 808, Yorktown Heights, NY 10598, 1-800-966-7522
American Institute of Cancer Research Newsletter, AICR, 1759 R Street NW, Washington, D.C., 20009 - free information and newsletter focusing on cancer and nutrition. Get on their mailing list by calling 1-800-843-8114. (free but donations appreciated!)
"Dr. Andrew Weil's Self Healing Newsletter"- 1-800-523-3296
"Environmental Nutrition" Newsletter- 1-800-829-5384
"Nutrition Action Health Letter", Center for Science in the Public Interest, Suite 300, 1875 Connecticut Ave., N.W., Washington, DC 20009-5728
"Vegetarian Nutrition and Health Letter", Loma Linda University, 1705 Nichol Hall, School of Public Health, Loma Linda, CA 92350
"Vegetarian Journal", Vegetarian Resource Group, PO Box 1463, Baltimore, MD 21203

All of these newsletters and others like them (Harvard, Mayo Clinic, UC-Berkeley, Tufts, Johns Hopkins, etc.) have a fee. Your local public library, medical system's patient education library, or even your own cancer center patient library may already subscribe to some of these so you could skim through them to look for articles of interest to you for free. In addition, there are certainly many additional informative newsletters for other cancer types.

I don't consider myself an "Internet Specialist", so I hesitate to make too many recommendations. It takes careful searching and lots of knowledge to *interpret* everything that is on the Internet. There are more "hits" on the Internet under the category "Alternative Medicine" than any other category, including many product marketing sites. In my opinion, these are some reliable places to start:

National Cancer Institute	http://wwwicic.nci.nih.gov
OncoLink (U of Penn)	http://www.oncolink.upenn.edu
American Institute for Cancer Research	http://www.aicr.org
NIH - Center of Alternative Medicine	http://altmed.od.nih.gov/nccam/
Office of Dietary Supplements	http://dietary-supplements.info.nih.gov
Tufts University Nutrition Navigator	http://navigator.tufts.edu
HealthWorld Online	http://www.healthy.net
Herb Research Foundation	http://www.herbs.org/herbs/
American Botanical Council	http://www.herbalgram.org
Center for Science in the Public Interest	http://www.cspinet.org
Alternative Medicine OnLine	http://altmedicine.com
CancerGuide	http://cancerguide.org
Alternative Medicine Sources	http://www.pitt.edu/~cbw/altm.html
BreastCancer.Net	http://wwwbreastcancer.net
Rosenthal Center for CAM	http://cpmcnet.columbia.edu:80/dept/rosenthal/
Medline (free access)	http://www.nlm.nih.gov/databases/freemedl.html

Moss, Ralph, Ph.D., *Alternative Medicine Online*, Equinox Press, 1997. A book to help you get started looking at sites for alternative medicine on the internet. I think about everything on the Internet very critically. Be cautious. *Think about who is funding the web site and the potential for bias in the presentation of information.*

For expert conduction and *interpretation* of an Internet search for an individual medical condition, I highly recommend the services of Health Decision Resources, Denise Jacob, RN, PhD, in Bloomfield Hills, MI, at 1-248-646-6659.

● *Miscellaneous*

National Cancer Institute – 1-800-4-CANCER – call for free information about cancer, educational materials, and clinical trials available for your type and stage of cancer.

National Coalition for Cancer Survivorship – 1-800-TOOLS-4-U – call for a free Cancer Survival Toolbox ™ containing 3 audio cassette tapes and workbook to help teach you self-advocacy skills as you prepare to participate in the fight for your life.

At least five journals devoted to alternative medicine and intended for MDs and other health care professionals have begun publication over the last couple of years. Check to see which are in the medical library of your doctor's hospital.

Alternative and Complementary Therapies, ed. Nicholas Gonzalez, MD
Alternative Medicine Journal, ed. Robert Enck, MD
Alternative Therapies in Health and Medicine, ed. Lawrence Dossey, MD
    (I buy this journal regularly at my local bookstore)
Journal of Alternative and Complementary Medicine, ed. Marc S. Micozzi, MD, PhD
Mental Medicine Update, ed. Robert Ornstein, PhD, and David Sobel, MD

"Living Dialogues" and "New Dimensions" shows on National Public Radio. Call your local public radio station to see if and what time these shows are aired in your locality.

Center for Alternative and Complementary Medicine (NIH) - 1-800-531-1794
Food and Drug Administration (FDA) "MedWatch" - to report adverse reactions to drugs or dietary supplements, including herbs - 1-800-332-1088 (you may call to "self-report")
The Herb Research Foundation operates a "Natural Healthcare Hotline" from which you may obtain information about herbs for a reasonable fee. Call 1-303-449-2265

The following four books are available with a study guide for CEUs for health care professionals from Helm Seminars and Publishing. For brochure and further info, call 940/497-3558 or Email kathy@helmnutrition.com

- Collinge, William, M.P.H., Ph.D., *The American Holistic Health Association Complete Guide to Alternative Medicine*, Warner Books, New York, 1996
- Tyler, Varro, Ph.D., Sc.D., *Herbs of Choice- The Therapeutic Use of Phytomedicinals*, Haworth Press, 1994
- Tyler, Varro, *The Honest Herbal: a Sensible Guide to the Use of Herbs and Related Remedies,* Pharmaceutical Products Press, New York, 3rd edition, 1993.
- Coughlin, CM, RD and RM DeBusk, RD, PhD, *Integrative Medicine: Your Quick Reference Guide,* Integrative Medicine, Inc., Tallahassee, FL 32315, 1997.

⚫ *Additional Helpful Books/Tapes*

Bender, Sue, *Plain and Simple: A Woman's Journey to the Amish,* Harper Collins Publisher, New York, 1989. The book that profoundly influenced me to listen to my heart and inner voice while I was making the difficult decision to leave my previous professional position in the ICU.

Benson, Herbert, MD, *Timeless Healing: The Power and Biology of Belief,* Simon and Schuster, New York, 1997. The author of *The Relaxation Response* and founder of Harvard Medical School's Mind/Body Institute summarizes all the current data and knowledge that shows the importance, value, and benefits of our beliefs for promoting healing. Easy and powerful reading.

Dossey, Larry, MD, *Healing Words: the Power of Prayer and the Practice of Medicine*, Harper Collins Publisher, 1993. I met Dr. Dossey and heard him speak in early April, 1998. I hung onto his every word during his presentations and feel totally comfortable recommending his books.

Dyer, Wayne, Ph.D., *Manifest Your Destiny: The Nine Spiritual Principles for Getting Everything You Want,* HarperCollins, New York, 1997. So far I have only listened to the tapes of this book. They were truly inspirational and left me tingling with goosebumps. These tapes (or the book) deserve to be a part of every cancer survivor's healing journey when she/he is ready to tackle the "what to do with the rest of my life" question.

Naparstek, Belleruth, guided imagery cassette tapes entitled "For People with Cancer" and "For People Undergoing Chemotherapy", Image Paths, Inc., 1-800-800-8661. I recently had the opportunity to meet Belleruth Naparstek and participate as she guided the audience through an imagery session at a conference. Even though I was 3 years past my last diagnosis at the time, and thought I finished done my healing, her imagery session was a profound experience and brought me even more healing. I highly recommend her tapes.

Siegel, Bernie, MD, many guided imagery and affirmation tapes available through his organization called ECaP. I have used several over the last 4 years and never fail to feel as though Bernie is actually holding my hand and telling me I can and will heal. These tapes have been very helpful. 1-800-700-8869.

Bartas, Jeanne. "Vegan Menu Items at Fast Food and Family-Style Restaurants, Part I." *Vegetarian Journal* Nov/Dec 1997. *http://www.vrg.org/journal/vj97nov/97bvegan.htm*

Bartas, Jeanne. "Vegan Menu Items at Fast Food and Family-Style Restaurants, Part II." *Vegetarian Journal* Jan/Feb 1998. *http://www.vrg.org/journal/vj98jan/981fast2.htm*

Bartas, Jeanne. "Vegetarian Menu Items at Restaurant and Quick Service Chains." Baltimore: The Vegetarian Resource Group, 1997. A condensed version is available on the vrg web site: http://www.vrg.org/nutshell/fast.htm Order info: Send $4.00 to The Vegetarian Resource Group (see address below) and request the "Guide to Fast Food."

Duyff, Roberta Larson, MS, RD, CFCS. ADA's Complete Food & Nutrition Guide. Chronimed Publishing: U.S., 1996, Chapter 15: "Your Food Away From Home" and pp. 567-9 ("Eating Out The Vegetarian Way").

Kurleto, Betsey, RD, MA & Price, Beverly, RD, MA. *Nutrition Secrets for Optimal Health.* Farmington Hills, Michigan: Tall Tree Publishing Company, 1996, pp. 172-175 ("Dining Out").

Havala, Suzanne, MS, RD. *Simple, Lowfat & Vegetarian.* Baltimore: The Vegetarian Resource Group, 1994.

Havala, Suzanne, MS, RD. *Good Foods, Bad Foods: What's Left to Eat?* Minneapolis: Chronimed Publishing, 1998. Chapter 10: "Eating Out" and Chapter 12: "Traveling Light."

Levy, Linda & Grabowski, Francine, MS, RD. *Low-Fat Living for Real People.* New York: Lake Isle Press, Inc., 1994, pp. 77-92 ("Strategies for Eating Out").

Messina, Virginia, MPH, RD & Messina, Mark, PhD. *The Vegetarian Way.* New York: Crown Trade Paperbacks, 1996, pp. 263-70 ("The Vegetarian Traveler").

Pensiero, Laura, RD, Oliveria, Susan, ScD, MPH, with Osborne, Michael, MD. *The Strang Cookbook for Cancer Prevention,* pp. 338-45. New York: Penguin Putnam, 1998.

Warshaw, Hope S., MMSc, RD, CDE. *The Restaurant Companion: A guide to healthier eating out.* Chicago: Surrey Books, Inc., 1995. (Updated version coming soon).

Wasserman, Debra & Stahler, Charles. *Meatless Meals for Working People.* Baltimore: The Vegetarian Resource Group, 1996, pp. 11-22 ("Eating Out").

American Institute for Cancer Research (AICR) - For pamphlets, call 1-800-843-8114 Cooking Solo (Meals on the Run section), Healthy Eating Away from Home

Dixie USA, Inc. Call 1-800-233-3668 to order Nutlettes Plus® cereal or other vegetarian products

Musk, Maye, MS, MS, RD, web page: www.mayemusk.com or e-mail mmusk@msn.com to request information on "nutritious food choices in restaurants."

The Vegetarian Resource Group - phone #: (410) 366-VEGE
Vegetarian Journal's Guide to Natural Foods Restaurants in the US and Canada
(To order, go to http://www.vrg.org/catalog/guide.htm or call above number)

Vegetarian Times magazine (often has information on finding vegetarian food abroad) To order, or for more information call (800) 435-9610

⚹ NOTES ⚹

❦ NOTES ❦

NOTES

🍎 NOTES 🍎

❦ ORDERING INFORMATION FOR ADDITIONAL BOOKS ❦

Additional copies of the 5th edition of *A Dietitian's Cancer Story* may be obtained by several different means.

- The book may be special ordered from any bookstore using the ISBN number: 0-9667238-1-3

- It is available for sale on the Internet at Amazon.com (www.Amazon.com) Search by my name or title. Amazon.com accepts charge cards.

- The book may also be ordered directly from me. Cost is $8.00/copy. Please add $2.00 s&h for the first copy and $1.00 s&h/copy for additional copies.
Michigan residents, please add $0.48 sales tax/copy. Thank you.
Canadian residents, please send $11.00/copy (US funds only).
Other countries, please send $12.00/copy (US funds only).

Please make checks or money orders payable to Diana Dyer and mail to the address listed below.

Bulk orders (10+) are priced lower. Please inquire for further information.

Last but not least, please visit my web site. I post great tasting, healthy recipes, "what's new", additional helpful web sites for cancer survivors, and occasionally, even have special pricing of my booklet.

Diana Dyer, MS, RD
PO Box 130221
Ann Arbor, MI 48113
Phone: 734-996-9260
Fax: 734-996-9262
Email: dianadyermsrd@provide.net
Web Site: www.dianadyermsrd.com

About the Author

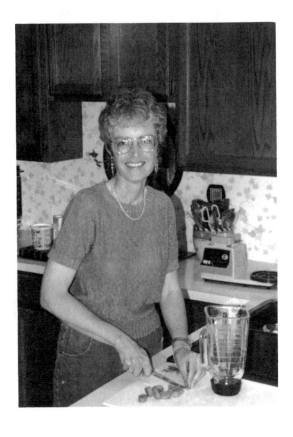

Diana Grant Dyer grew up in Toledo, Ohio. Her neuroblastoma was treated at The Toledo Hospital, Toledo, OH, and her two breast cancers were treated at Evanston Hospital, Evanston, IL, and The University of Michigan's Comprehensive Cancer Center, Ann Arbor, MI.

She received her B.S. degree in Biology from Purdue University. Her M.S. degree in Nutritional Sciences and Dietetic Internship were completed at The University of Wisconsin and The University of Wisconsin Hospitals, respectively. In between cancer diagnoses, she has spent her entire career as a dietitian working at several hospitals in the Midwest, specializing in nutritional care for the critically ill patient.

Diana currently has a private practice focusing solely on coaching people with a cancer diagnosis about diet and lifestyle changes to optimize therapy and recovery of the mind, body, and spirit. She is available for both private consultations in Ann Arbor, Michigan, and telephone consults.

Diana is a frequently requested speaker for professional, patient, and public groups, speaking on her cancer story and "integrated" recovery path. In addition, Diana has been interviewed on national TV (MSNBC) and has multiple newspaper, radio, TV, and Internet interviews.

Diana was honored in May, 1998, by The Michigan Dietetic Association with its Individual Public Relations Award. This award is given annually to the dietitian in Michigan who has done the most during the previous year to increase the visibility and the professional stature of the Registered Dietitian as the nutrition expert to the general public.

Diana lives in Ann Arbor, Michigan, with her wonderful husband Dick, terrific sons Eric and Garrison, two adoring cats Tiger and Panther, and assorted other critters including her backyard birds. Friends continue trying to teach her how to quilt, but her passions are Scottish fiddle music and birding.